M000211813

"*Nearly Departed* is a tribute to all of us who are trying to live this messy thing called life, and all the surprising beauty you can find within. Few authors can move you to tears with their words—Gila is one of them. Reading this book, I felt like she was my best friend telling me her story, describing the details with joy and faithfulness, and pulling me in and never letting go."
—**Sarah Cooper, comedian and author of** *Foolish*

"Pfeffer seamlessly blends tears and laughter in her vibrant debut memoir. . . . The results are as funny as they are heartfelt and inspiring."—***Publishers Weekly***

"*Nearly Departed* is a book about loss, grief, and mortality that nonetheless sparkles with joy. And it is very, very funny. In fact, the darker it got, the more I laughed, which is how you know it was written by a Jew. I loved it."
—**Catherine Newman, author of**
We All Want Impossible Things

"Bringing humor to tragedy is a tightrope act, but Gila does it beautifully. Her writing is compelling and contains an irresistible combination of depth and lightness."
—**Wendi Aarons, author of** *I'm Wearing Tunics Now*

"After her mom's death upended her family, Gila was forced to take control of her own destiny in order to protect herself and the people she loved. A rallying cry for prevention, Pfeffer shows off her gift for turning tragedy, grief, and loss into something to laugh about."
—**Emi Nietfeld, author of** *Acceptance*

nearly departed

A Memoir

Adventures in Loss, Cancer, and Other Inconveniences

gila pfeffer

THE EXPERIMENT

NEW YORK

The Experiment, LLC I 220 East 23rd Street, Suite 600 I New York, NY 10010-4658
theexperimentpublishing.com

This book is a memoir and contains the reflections, opinions, and ideas of its author. Some names and characteristics have been changed, some events have been compressed, and some dialogue has been recreated. It is sold with the understanding that the author and publisher are not engaged in rendering medical, health, or any other kind of personal and/or professional services in the book. The author and publisher specifically disclaim all responsibility for any liability, loss, or risk—personal or otherwise—that is incurred as a consequence, directly or indirectly, of the use and application of any of the contents of this book.

THE EXPERIMENT and its colophon are registered trademarks of The Experiment, LLC. Many of the designations used by manufacturers and sellers to distinguish their products are claimed as trademarks. Where those designations appear in this book and The Experiment was aware of a trademark claim, the designations have been capitalized.

The Experiment's books are available at special discounts when purchased in bulk for premiums and sales promotions as well as for fund-raising or educational use. For details, contact us at info@theexperimentpublishing.com.

Library of Congress Cataloging-in-Publication Data

Names: Pfeffer, Gila, author.
Title: Nearly departed : adventures in loss, cancer, and other
   inconveniences : a memoir / Gila Pfeffer.
Description: New York : The Experiment, [2024]
Identifiers: LCCN 2024013723 (print) I LCCN 2024013724 (ebook) I ISBN
   9781891011627 (hardcover) I ISBN 9781891011634 (ebook)
Subjects: LCSH: Pfeffer, Gila. I Cancer--Patients--United
   States--Biography. I Children of cancer patients--United
   States--Biography. I Jewish women--United States--Biography. I
   Cancer--Genetic aspects.
Classification: LCC RC265.6.P474 A3 2024 (print) I LCC RC265.6.P474
   (ebook) I DDC 616.99/40092 [B]--dc23/eng/20240506
LC record available at https://lccn.loc.gov/2024013723
LC ebook record available at https://lccn.loc.gov/2024013724

ISBN 978-1-891011-62-7
Ebook ISBN 978-1-891011-63-4

Jacket and text design, and cover photograph, by Beth Bugler
Author photograph by Sarah Raanan

Manufactured in the United States of America

First printing July 2024
10 9 8 7 6 5 4 3 2 1

For Phil, who keeps his promises

And for Ezra, Lea, Tani, and Kivi, who saved my life

Contents

Author's Note

A memoir is a nonfiction narrative based on the author's personal memories. In writing this story, I relied on my own memories as well as firsthand accounts of friends and family. Those, by definition, are subjective. Some minor details have been changed, as have some names and identities, so if you think I'm writing about you, you may be right, but we'll never know for sure. There are so many people who played a vital role in seeing me through difficult times and I'd have loved to have written about every single one of you, but my editor said I couldn't write an eight-hundred-page book; I'm not Barbra Streisand.

One often meets his destiny on the road he takes to avoid it.

—Grand Master Oogway, *Kung Fu Panda*

Yom asal, yom basal ("One day honey, one day onions")

—Old Arabic proverb

INTAKE FORM

One thing no one ever tells you about being an adult is how much time you'll spend filling out forms. The simple act of existing requires a preposterous amount of paperwork. Broadly speaking, forms fall into one of two categories: the kind you can complete at home (e.g., insurance claims, anything school and camp related, online returns where you have to choose the code that best describes the reason you're not keeping the silver sequined jeans you imagined would look as chic on you as they did on the model) and the ones you are handed in a waiting room (e.g., the medical variety). Waiting to be seen by your health care provider is boring at best, anxiety inducing at worst, so answering a bunch of personal questions is as much about communicating your medical history to a new practitioner as it is an activity to pass the time; the adult equivalent of handing a child a coloring book. It also functions as a pleasant stroll down memory lane, a scrapbook, if you will, of your medical history. An added bonus: Holding a clipboard like you're a club bouncer checking names on the VIP list feels cool.

Why not just pull out my smartphone and partake in an endless buffet of streaming content, online news outlets, or social media posts to stave off the boredom, you ask? Because it is 2006 and there is no Netflix or any other streaming, no Wi-Fi, no Instagram. We barely even have texting. My Motorola flip phone does precisely one thing—calls people—and it rests in my pleather handbag while I sit in the fluorescent-lit reception area of a hospital near my home in New Jersey.

I'm thirty-two years old and here for my first-ever breast MRI. You would be here, too, if you had my family's history of cancer. By thirty, I was the oldest living member of my family. It was also the age at which I had my first mammogram. My ob-gyn and a breast specialist advised me to start screening when I was ten years younger than my closest relative was when she was diagnosed with breast cancer—in this case, my mom. She was forty and died less than two years later. My health insurance provider, however, disagreed and told me they wouldn't cover a mammogram until I was forty. I told them, "Without a mammogram, I'll be dead by forty."

Since that baseline screening, I've had two more mammograms and a third baby. My husband Phil and I have decided to try for baby number four, but now I'm inching closer toward my mother's age of diagnosis, my doctors have strongly advised I first add a breast ultrasound and MRI to my prevention roster. We have to be extra sure nothing is lurking in my mammaries before embarking on a fourth and final pregnancy.

The receptionist hands me a clipboard with a double-sided questionnaire and apologizes; they are running late.

"No problem," I say, hoping I sound nonchalant. "I've got plenty to keep myself occupied." I've never had any kind of MRI before, and I'm nervous. I return to my seat and prepare to indulge in my three favorite waiting-room activities:

1. Being alone with my thoughts.

2. Purging my handbag of old receipts, Kit Kat wrappers, and wadded-up tissues used to wipe my kids' noses. (This activity pairs well with #1.)

3. Filling out the "Have you ever had any of the following diseases?" portion of the intake form.

It's like taking a test I know I'll ace. With rapid-fire flicks of a pen, I make my way down the "no" column, never once having to make a mark in a "yes" box. "Yes" is the domain of the sick and, unlike my parents and grandparents, disease has not yet come for me.

Have you ever had any of the following?

Heart disease: Nope

Hypertension: No, ma'am.

IBS: Thankfully no. Miraculous considering its high incidence among Ashkenazi Jews.

Rheumatoid arthritis? Osteoporosis? Joint pain? Not this healthy filly!

Cancer: I was hoping you'd ask because this is, by far, my favorite question to answer with an emphatic, dramatic, and cinematic *no*.

This is my own twisted version of "Never Have I Ever." Although my life is hardly problem-free, I've always been healthy—no small feat in my family. I know firsthand what happens when, instead of preempting a problem, you wait for the problem to find you.

The reason I've filled out so many medical forms in so many medical offices in my twenties and early thirties is not because I am sick. Quite the opposite. I am doing my damndest to avoid illness. And when I say illness, I mean cancer.

Do you have a family history of breast cancer? Do I ever!

Which side of the family? Both! We are an equal opportunity breast cancer conglomerate.

If yes, which family members? Here's a table for your convenience:

RELATIVE	CURRENT AGE, IF LIVING	AGE AT DEATH, IF DECEASED	HISTORY OF CANCER TYPE	AGE AT CANCER DIAGNOSIS
Mother		42	Breast	40
Maternal Grandmother		49	Breast & Ovarian	40
Great Aunt		50-something	Breast	Not sure
Paternal Grandmother		70-something Died of heart disease	Breast	Not sure, but survived

Do you have a history of other cancers? Yes! I feel like I'm winning this game. Will there be prizes?

Which side of the family? My father died of colon cancer when he was fifty-four. Many of my relatives were murdered in the Holocaust and my grandparents—who survived—are no longer living either, so there's a big, gaping hole in our family medical history. There's no one left to ask these questions. We work with what we've got.

By now, I've grown accustomed to doctors and nurses skimming over my completed form, their eyes widening, giving an incredulous shake of the head, which means they'd arrived at the portion devoted to my family history. I've come to recognize their looks of surprise and tenderness layered with acknowledgment and topped with a glaze of admiration for someone who learned the hard way about the importance of preventative medicine. I'd be lying if I said I don't enjoy the kudos.

Did you breastfeed? Yes, but I struggled with it and stopped after a few months per child. My main motivation was the fact that breastfeeding has been found to reduce the risk of breast cancer.

Have you been having regular mammograms? How often? Yes, annually since I turned thirty, but let me tell you, I had to fight for that first one.

Please indicate any breast symptoms you're currently experiencing:

Mass or Lump ☐   **Nipple Discharge** ☐
Skin Changes ☐   **Breast Pain** ☐

Other: I don't wait for symptoms before going for preventative screenings. Symptoms = you're too late.

Do you have any mental health issues? I mean, my parents both died young leaving nothing behind but debt and a little sister to raise, so, yeah, I probably have mental health issues, but who's got time to address those? I saw a therapist a few times after my mom died and then a few more times after my dad died, so that ought to tide me over for the rest of my life, or at least endow me with the fortitude to crush my anxiety like a grape and bury it in the least accessible parts of myself. Sorry, what was the question again?

"Mrs. Pfeffer?" A technician in pink scrubs appears and searches the waiting room, her eyes finally landing on me. I gather up my debris-free purse and coat. "Sorry to have kept you waiting, it's been crazy today! Follow me and we'll get you into a changing room."

I stow my belongings in an assigned locker and change into a pink (ugh) seersucker wraparound gown. Slipping the plastic bracelet onto my wrist, I step out into the mauve (barf) linoleum-tiled corridor and consider the technician's words: "It's been crazy today." I hope my case is one of her boring ones. In medical terms, boring is good. Boring is safe.

She leads me into the enclosure, points to a table with cereal-bowl-size holes in it, and instructs me to lie face down, positioning my breasts through the openings. She hands me a pair of earplugs and asks if I'd like any particular type of music played during my scan to keep me relaxed—it's critical that I don't move while the machine is scanning my breasts.

"No music, thanks," I say, "I'll probably just fall asleep in there anyway."

"I hear you, I'm a mom, too," she confides, and we chuckle at the fact that even the most invasive medical procedures are opportunities for an uninterrupted nap, but I'm not even kidding; I absolutely would 100 percent fall asleep in that claustrophobia-inducing tube because I've been tired since 2001 when my first son was born.

The technician covers me with a pink (dear God make it stop) blanket before retreating to her glass booth overlooking the MRI enclosure. Picturing what my boobs must look like from underneath—two pendulous socks weighed down by oranges—makes me laugh.

"Ready?" the technician's voice comes through the microphone all muffled, tinny, distant. Keeping my head down, I raise one hand and give a thumbs-up. My tray table starts to slide forward until I am fully encased in the greige tube. I fall asleep almost immediately. It takes three people to repeat my name and gently but determinedly shake my shoulders to wake me up when the scan is over. I can't remember when I last slept that well.

A week later, the scan results are in: all clear. Phil and I can now forge ahead with the production of a younger sibling for our two sons and daughter, safe in the knowledge that I've been given a clean bill of health.

Ever since my mother died, I've been consistently following the same prevention protocol: check, double-check, get on with the business of living, and then check some more. I will keep harm at bay, never allowing it the chance to gain purchase on my body by never, not for one second, letting my guard down.

1

another motherless daughter

The first indication that my mother might have breast cancer came as I was boarding a plane to Israel for a semester abroad. I was eighteen years old.

I stood in the departures zone at JFK airport, clustered with my parents and three younger sisters, like many other families who'd come to see their kids off for a year of post–high school study in a Jerusalem seminary. In my case, it was half a year. I'd already spent the previous one studying and touring the land, as is customary for Orthodox Jewish students the year after high school. It was early September 1992, and the plan was to be back by January and enrolled at a New York City university.

"Boy, I would give my left arm to trade places with you," my dad said. He was fond of American figures of speech even though they sometimes sounded off-kilter when spoken in his faint Hungarian accent. He clutched my face between his slight, smooth hands, and held my gaze, his lower lids barely containing a pool of tears. "Make sure you put in a good word for me with the Big Man at the Wall, OK?" Although my father was a deeply religious man who prayed three times each day, he hoped my prayers at the holiest place on earth might reverse his yearslong financial decline. Here he was, asking his oldest daughter to include a request that he miraculously find his way out of debt while praying to God at the Western Wall in Jerusalem, a city he dreamed of living in. The embarrassment in his voice made me wince.

"Sure, Ta, of course," I promised. It was what he needed to hear. We half hugged in the awkward way of two people who are emotionally constipated, and I moved on to my petite mom who had my baby sister, Gita, clamped onto her hip. She seemed distracted, jittery, repeatedly tucking a strand of permed, bottle-blonde hair behind one ear. Perhaps she was preoccupied by the probability that I'd return from my half-gap year the way I'd returned from my full one: thirty pounds heavier and without any marriage prospects. Sensing her dread, I enveloped her and the baby in a tight hug, planted a few extra kisses on Gita's fat rosy cheeks, and stage-whispered to my mom, "Don't worry, Ma, I won't gain weight again." (Narrator: Gila did gain weight again.)

"Oh, I'm not worried about that, Mamaleh, it all came off when you came home last time. Just remember to write lots of letters and if you have to call home, keep it short. International calls are *so* expensive!" Maybe if I prayed hard enough at the Wall, I'd be able to collect call like the rest of my friends and have a conversation that lasted more than two minutes.

"I know, Ma. I'll write. Make sure to send lots of photos of Gita-Pita." Turning to Miryam and Rivky, I said, "You guys had better write to me and I promise to write back, OK? I'll see if I can fit an Egozi bar in the envelope." Egozi bars were my favorite Israeli candy bar. Nodding enthusiastically, they promised they would write and I gave them each a lingering hug and kiss before pulling away, eager to board my plane. The only family member not present was my seventeen-year-old brother Eli, which was just as well; our interactions mainly included pranking each other, name calling, and that one time he accidentally broke my toe when I was nine. That was our love language.

Other passengers, most of whom were around my age, were saying their last goodbyes and heading toward the gate a few feet away. This was back when your family could walk you all the way to the gate rather than leave you at the end of a long security line. Good times.

"Faigie, I'll take the girls to the car and wait for you there while you, uh, finish saying goodbye," my father told my mother, waving at me as he and my sisters turned to head back to the parking lot. My mother stood there frozen, in a pink, satin-trimmed sweatshirt, gripping Gita with both arms. Her eyes darted from side to side while her mouth kept opening and clamping shut.

"Bye, Gi. I love you!" she finally managed. Her voice sounded foreign as it produced a phrase seldom used between us. My mother and I had struggled to understand each other, almost from the moment I entered my teens. She had little kids to tend to and a household to manage on an ever-decreasing budget. I wanted to be with my friends, she wanted me home to babysit a growing roster of siblings. We both lacked the capacity to engage in emotionally honest conversations and most of our attempts ended with me storming off to my room. A first-generation American and the daughter of Holocaust survivors, my mother was well-versed in frugality, but not child psychology. Plus, I was not an easy firstborn to cut her teeth on. I was moody, cynical, unsure of how the world worked, and desperately in need of unconditional love and acceptance.

The "I love you" landed like a record scratch. *Of course* she loved me, but couldn't she stick to showing it by baking my favorite marble Bundt cake, fixing the hem of my skirt on her sewing machine, and letting me borrow the minivan when I wanted to drive to my friends in Brooklyn? We could, maybe, take our relationship to the "I love you" phase in the future, but JFK airport was not the place to undergo a rebrand. I was already halfway to the gate and awkwardly turned around to repeat it back to her.

"I love you too, Ma." I said it as quietly as possible, hoisting my overstuffed duffel bag onto my shoulder, and with a final wave to Gita, turned back to join the line forming at the gate. Looking around at the other sniffly families who were getting in one last hug or group photo, I was relieved our goodbye was over. My parents and I weren't mushy. The main emotions I experienced as a teenager were angst, confusion, and the sense that I had to get out of Staten Island as quickly as possible.

With only a few passengers standing between me and passport control, I was nearly home free when I heard my name being called from a few feet away. Loudly. In front of everybody.

"Gila!" It was my mom. Of course. But now she was crying. Making a scene. A scene that I'd have been better equipped to handle five minutes earlier when I was standing right next to her. This display of emotion was remarkably off-brand for her. It was disconcerting.

"Gi!" I turned toward her. My insides were simultaneously on fire and frozen, like what I imagine that muscle-soothing cream Icy Hot must feel like.

"I think I might have breast cancer!" She didn't quite shout the words, but she didn't whisper them, either. I was equal parts self-conscious and mortified, and the sound of her crying was immediately overtaken by a high-pitched ringing in my ears. If anyone else heard what she said, I couldn't tell. There were tearful parents everywhere seeing their kids off, so despite the drama of the moment, anyone may have thought she was just really sad to see me go.

She was sobbing now, looking at me across knots of people as if I'd know the right thing to say because I was her eldest child and she had no sisters and her mother died at forty-nine of a disease she now thought she had, and that she probably wanted to find out the results of whatever tests before laying this piece of news on me, but watching her daughter walk away and leave her alone with a house full of kids and a husband who'd been struggling to make ends meet for years had made her panic—and she could no longer contain her terror or her hunch that it is 100 percent going to be breast cancer because her mom's half-sister died of it, too, and although this was well before anyone knew what genetic testing was, it didn't take a PhD in biology to know that breast cancer ran in our family.

I could have asked *why* she thought she might have cancer. I could have said, "What are you talking about?" as I imagine most people would have.

But I had no words. What I *did* have was an overwhelming urge to board that plane, the sooner the better. I wanted to get away from a household where my relationships with my friends and my need for sleep were undervalued, where financial problems and the arguments they caused went from bad to worse, where I increasingly suspected I might be better at life than my parents who couldn't seem to get their act together. Here, in the airport, was one more example of my parents mishandling a bombshell that another family might have dropped with greater care. And better timing.

I faced her but didn't move. I knew I was supposed to say something, but it had to be the *right* thing, something to reassure my mother while also not requiring me to forgo my plans. I didn't make a sound. This wasn't my family's first time at the terrible news rodeo, and I knew how things would go. She would 100 percent, for sure, have cancer. Right there, in the airport, I started to brace myself for my mother's death.

Whether it was shock or self-preservation or a little bit of both, I pivoted on my heel, shifted my duffel to the other shoulder, and, along with a gaggle of girls my age, headed through the gate to board my plane, wishing I'd said something or, better still, that she'd said nothing.

Two weeks later, my six roommates and I sat around the tiny kitchen table in the Jerusalem apartment we shared. Like me, they'd come back for a second year of study. The seven of us shared one shower that produced hot water only if you thought far enough in advance to switch on the solar panel, two poorly insulated bedrooms, and Jurassic-era kitchen appliances, but it was ours for the semester and we loved it. A beige plastic telephone bolted to the kitchen wall was for incoming calls only. When I'd last called home a day after landing safely, it was from a pay phone around the corner. It was my father who'd answered. "We're still waiting to hear from the doctor, Mamaleh," he said.

My friends and I were laughing about someone's failed attempt at a lasagna when the phone rang. Rachel, my childhood next-door neighbor, answered it with a theatrical "Hellllooooooooooo," but her face quickly fell, and she looked at me. My hands shook as she passed me the receiver.

The girls crowded around me, unsure of what to do as my body crumpled and I shook from sobbing so hard. My mother's wailing blew like a trumpet through the phone and my friends began to cry, too. I was so sad and so scared but oddly relieved; now, I wouldn't have to wonder anymore. I'd long assumed that cancer would come for her the way it had for her mother and aunt. That's what cancer does. It comes for you. How was I supposed to know that it was possible to survive cancer if I'd never witnessed any family member do it? What I couldn't understand is how I'd seen it coming and she hadn't.

A tidal wave of terms I didn't understand issued forth from my mother's mouth. I had no way, in a pre-internet world, of investigating them. She said, "suspicious mass"; she said "mammogram" and "chemo" and "radical mastectomy" (the word "mastectomy" is alarming enough without adding the foaming-at-the-mouth "radical"). I realized then that when my father asked me to "put in a good word at the Wall," he was referring to more than just his debts.

"Do you want me to fly home early, Mommy? I will if you want me to." I hoped she'd say no.

"No, sweetheart," she whispered, her voice wet and thick. "They're going to do a biopsy"—another word I didn't know— "and we'll see what we're dealing with. Anyway, it's only a few months until December. You enjoy your time there." I suspected she really did want me to come home, to have at least one more adult(ish) around. She hadn't been much older than me when her own mother died of breast and ovarian cancer, and I wondered what their interactions had been like in the years leading up to her death. It was something we'd never discussed and not something I felt comfortable asking.

"OK, Ma," I sniffled, "I'll daven extra hard for you at the Kotel, and I'll be home before you know it. You're going to be OK; I know it. You *have* to be OK, for us and especially Gita-Pita." I meant it about praying for her at the Wall. Not so much the part about being OK. But it was what she needed to hear, and it was all I had to offer from so far away. Over the next few years, in the name of bringing her comfort, I would say lots of things to my mother that I didn't mean. We both would.

"I hope you're right," she mumbled while blowing her nose. I heard Gita's voice calling out for her in the background and felt a pang of homesickness. "I'm going to go now, Mamaleh, this phone call is getting very expensive."

———

Chanukah came and went with all of its donuts and latkes and menorah-lighting parties, which I attended with the other students on my program. The occasion also served as a farewell to the second-year crew; it was time for us to go home. I spent the twelve-hour flight seated next to my best friend Suri, who in a few weeks' time would also be my college roommate. She bopped her head in time to "Baby Got Back" by Sir Mix-a-Lot, while I, Walkman-less, tried to dodge the dread that was burrowing its way into every cell. I didn't know what I was coming home to but, based on updates I'd been getting from my parents over (short) phone calls, and what my friends had been hearing from their parents, I knew things at home were dire. In early November, after putting it off for a month, my mother had finally had a biopsy. It showed a large, poorly differentiated infiltrating ductal carcinoma, meaning the cancer started in her milk ducts and spread to nearby tissue. Later that month, she began a grueling regimen of chemotherapy that went on until January. I'd be coming home at the tail end of her treatment and when I tried to imagine what she might look like, my brain could conjure nothing other than Deborah Winger in *Terms of Endearment*. Suri and I'd obsessively watched the film on her VCR during our senior year. Often we'd fast-forward to the final few scenes and bawl our eyes out watching Winger say goodbye to her two young sons.

My father was waiting for me in the arrivals terminal at JFK wearing his standard uniform: tan chinos, a white button-down shirt, and thin pleather windbreaker. We rode home in our stale-smelling Dodge Caravan, or as my friends jokingly referred to it, "The Toaster on Wheels." The radio was set to 1010 WINS lest we miss a vital traffic update, and between chitchat about my time away, how much Gita had grown, and how brave Miryam and Rivky had been, my dad doled out tidbits on my mother's current state.

"She's a fighter, your mother," he said, looking ahead at the road while providing me with no new information. Everyone undergoing cancer treatment was referred to as a "fighter." I learned that from watching movies.

"She's doing this crazy macrobiotic diet. She thinks it will stop the cancer from growing bigger." He shrugged. "I don't know, maybe it will work. Maybe *Hashem Yisbarach* will make it work," he said, invoking one of God's many names. "You know how Mommy is. She still takes those homeopathy pills, too." For years, my mother had tried to get our family to shun Western medicine in favor of homeopathy. At one point, she'd had ambitions to become a homeopath herself and bought a blue plastic tool kit filled with ChapStick-size vials full of sweet, white pellets that were supposed to cure our headaches and nausea, warts and period cramps. My family took to this the same way we took to her trying to introduce tofu into our diets: We didn't.

"How does she look?" I asked, even though I'd be seeing her soon. Maybe a few concrete details would help me move past the Debra Winger image and onto something resembling my mom.

"She's tiny, so skinny, and she wears a hat these days." He started to say something more, then stopped, took a breath, and started again. "The insurance company has been terrible. The bills, Gi, they're astronomical." He slumped over the wheel, and I could see his eyes welling up. My prayers at the Kotel didn't seem to have worked. We pulled into the garage and as the electronic door lowered behind us, I felt a little queasy. My father unloaded my suitcase and I headed into the house, forcing myself to smile brightly for my mother.

We hugged hello in our mauve-tiled kitchen where she stood wearing an oversize sweater that was also mauve. She really loved mauve. The chemotherapy was potent. It had transformed her into a Shrinky-Dink version of herself: gaunt, discolored, translucent. It was like hugging a cardboard cut-out, all bony angles. As I pulled away, I could see her eyebrows were gone, replaced by penciled arches. Aside from her shining brown eyes and signature red lacquered nails, she was unrecognizable.

Faigie Reinitz, nee Lerner, had always been petite, her outsize post-birth hips disproportionate to her slender wrists, calves, and ankles, all of which she'd passed down to me. As a newly married Orthodox Jewish woman, she'd covered her hair with wigs and scarves as was customary in her community, but had abandoned the practice long before I was old enough to remember. The mom I knew permed her mousy brown hair in the early eighties and started frosting it with blonde tips toward the end of the decade. By 1990, she'd gone layered honey blonde and that was her last hairstyle before she lost it all to chemo.

I pulled away and said, "Hi, Ma." And then a partial truth, "It's good to be home."

"You look great, Gi!" she lied, choosing to ignore the fact that I'd come home from Israel a bit chunky. Again. She'd spent money we didn't have to get me braces when I was thirteen to improve my chances of bagging a husband later on, and there I was, sabotaging her efforts.

She pulled gently at the straw-like remnants of her bleached hair peeking out from under a bucket hat and blinked back tears. My mother had always been pretty with good cheekbones to offset her sharp nose and small chin. Without any cosmetic intervention, she looked ten years younger than she was. Now I was home, there was one more witness to her decrepitude.

"I'm so happy you're home, ma-ma." For as long as I could remember, she had called me some version of "little mother." Ma-ma. Mamaleh. A terrible thought occurred to me: I'll have to be more than just a little mother soon.

Miryam, Rivky, and Gita came running into the kitchen screeching, "Gi! Gi!" and welcomed me home with hugs and stories about the shenanigans they'd been up to in my absence. It was the relief I needed from my dark thoughts. They looked the same as when I'd left them at JFK and that was a huge comfort. If I focused on them, I could almost trick myself into believing everything was fine.

My parents and I agreed I should move into my college dorm in Manhattan as planned, rather than drop anchor back in my childhood bedroom. "You'll have a better chance of being set up on dates and meeting a good shidduch," my mother reasoned. As much as she'd have loved an extra driver and pair of hands around the house while finishing the last of her chemo, the fact was I was weeks away from my nineteenth birthday, which, according to many in our community, meant I was ready to start seriously considering marriage.

Nothing about me said "ready for marriage." I hadn't started college, hadn't yet figured out who I was, and wasn't financially self-sufficient—being able to support myself before considering marriage was nonnegotiable. I didn't know how to book my own airline ticket, carve a roasted chicken (which would require me to first know how to roast a chicken), or even what music genres I liked. If asked, I'd have answered with "Anything they play on 95.5 WPLJ" because I didn't know where or how else to find music.

"You could meet a nice YU boy," she continued dreamily, refer-ring to the boys at the Jewish all-male campus farther uptown from my all-women's Stern College campus in Midtown Manhattan. The separate campuses were part of what attracted religious Jews to Yeshiva University, a natural next step for students coming from same-sex Orthodox Jewish high schools. Although I'd been accepted at my mother's alma mater, the Fashion Institute of Technology, to pursue one of my dreams of becoming a fashion designer, I'd panicked at the last minute when I realized I wouldn't be able to afford the housing and would have to live at home. Stern College for Women aggressively recruited students like me who'd attended Yeshiva high schools, and offered enticing scholarships.

"Ma, please. I'm not ready to get married, OK?"

"But if you met a nice Jewish boy . . . one who could take care of you . . ."

"I'll take care of myself. Ugh, stop."

"I just don't want your life to be so hard." She stopped short of saying "like mine is."

Whether she intuited that she had less time left on this earth than her peers, or was simply looking for some joy in her life, my mother's singular focus when it came to me was marrying "well." Not my education, not my career potential, not even breast cancer, which clearly runs in our family, and how to avoid it.

Because of my three semesters in Israel, I entered college as an upper sophomore majoring in English literature while also doing office jobs found in want ads. I needed the cash; my dad had none to give me. I went home most weekends to spend Shabbat with my family, to be the cool big sister home from the big city. I felt better suited at playing a cameo role than the witness I'd become to my mother's decline, her newfound confidante and repository for her worst fears and greatest sorrows.

The chemo worked better than expected and my mother's tumor shrank considerably. From what I could gather by eavesdropping on several conversations between my parents (the bedroom doors in our house were like wafers), she'd been advised to have an immediate radical mastectomy. My mother didn't want a mastectomy. She convinced herself she didn't need one, even though a medically trained specialist warned that her tumor could and likely would grow back, bigger and resistant to chemotherapy. I was convinced that she was making a terrible mistake.

Instead, she prescribed herself a never-ending stream of alternative "remedies." In no particular order (and sometimes simultaneously) she tried the following.

A detox soak: This involved sitting on an upturned bucket in our family bathtub while her tiny feet soaked in a basin filled with purple dye.

A macrobiotic diet: During chemo, my mom subsisted on a steady diet of Ensure, a pasty, calorie-dense drink that came in chocolate, vanilla, and strawberry flavors. (I tasted all three and can report that they were not half bad. Or maybe they were terrible, but we never had any good snacks in our house. To me, they tasted like milkshakes.) She'd read somewhere that a macrobiotic diet could fight cancer as it cut out processed foods, sugar, eggs, dairy, and even some vegetables. Eager to help, her friend Elaine bought a macrobiotic cookbook and prepared a steady stream of meals. The "bird food" as my father called it was unappealing to my chocaholic mother, and she often opted out of eating altogether.

Homeopathic remedies: Long before her diagnosis, my mother had befriended a homeopath whose cure for everything was placing tiny, sweet white pellets with names like Ptoojah, Arnica, and Nux Vomica (which inspired endless vomit jokes among my siblings) under your tongue. After studying homeopathy (reading one book), she bought a kit of her own and confidently dispensed the candies—uh, remedies—to cure our headaches, menstrual cramps, and stubbed toes. By the time she got sick, she was well-versed in which pellets would pair best with her macrobiotic buckwheat groats stir-fry.

Shark cartilage: That's right, SHARK CARTILAGE. It became a popular medicine in the seventies for things like osteoarthritis, psoriasis, and . . . *cancer*, three conditions that naturally go hand in hand. Someone somewhere had noted that sharks don't get cancer so eating their cartilage (in pill form) could prevent humans from getting it. My mom was undergoing treatment in the early nineties, which just goes to show how skilled the shark cartilage manufacturers' marketing departments were, keeping this stupidity going for more than two decades.

A special machine, of which there was only one in the world, which sCIenTiSTs invented to SUCK THE CANCER OUT OF YOUR BODY. OK, she didn't actually try this one because it was a financial and logistical no-go, but she sure wanted to. Lord knows where she learned of this "treatment," but she got her hands on a VHS tape and we all gathered around the TV to watch a grainy video of a man who looked "very sick" get connected to a sort of HVAC duct, which was attached to a riveted, metal contraption that looked like a prop from a 1950s sci-fi movie. The machine made loud suction noises as the man's torso was pulled in and out of the duct, which resulted in some beige, fatty globs oozing out of the machine through a funnel and into a bucket. The movie *Man on the Moon* wouldn't come out until six years later, but it contains an eerily similar scene. It tells the story of comedian Andy Kaufman (as played by Jim Carrey) who visits a healer in a desperate attempt to cure his terminal cancer. He observes the healer reach into a bucket of bloody prawns, one of which he conceals in his fist to create the illusion of "pulling the disease" out of Kaufman who lies pale and bald on a table, laughing at himself for falling for the very sort of trick he would famously play on his audiences.

The tinctures and infomercial-style remedies were bad enough but the cancer-be-gone machine—which was in Russia, by the way—was at a level of absurdity I couldn't handle.

"Ma!" I yelled on a weekend visit home, "It's a scam! If any of this actually cured cancer, it would already be available here in the US!"

My mother was sold. I was horrified.

She found her way to all of these alternative therapies in a pre-internet era. I can only imagine the sort of hoaxes she'd have been roped into had she had access to Facebook. If turning her feet purple was a supplement to traditional Western medical treatments, it might not have been a bad thing, but she turned to them *instead* of undergoing the mastectomy her doctors were begging her to have.

It would be years—and many readings of her medical charts—until I was able to fully grasp the deadly choice she made. In a letter dated January 6, 1994, her radiologist wrote to her breast cancer surgeon, which, like many inter-doctor letters do, opened with a recap of my mom's journey so far: "This (chemotherapy) was done between November and January 1993 with apparently excellent response. She was supposed to have a mastectomy then but apparently she refused, and chemotherapy was continued."

And while she was soaking her feet in purple dye, picking at sautéed rice noodles with tempeh, and ingesting a shark's actual weight in pills, her tumor had the opportunity to grow to eight centimeters, larger and more invasive than it was before. It was now the size of an orange and had spread to many of her lymph nodes.

By May 1993, she finally agreed to have her left breast and surrounding tissue fully removed, but she'd missed her chance; the cancer was too big and far-reaching for a mastectomy. She needed more chemo first. By the time she became eligible for the surgery again that September, the toxic cocktail of drugs had left her looking like a skeletal ghost. Her skin was gray, her mouth filmy, and she no longer bothered covering her bald head. I was embarrassed by how excruciating it was to look at her. It was the start of my junior year in college and I couldn't move into the dorm fast enough.

I was keenly aware of her despair over my failure to find a suitor, despite her persistent conspiring with our local match-maker to set me up on blind dates. The dates were awkward and draining, but I agreed to them as an act of mercy for my mother. There was little else I could do for her.

On September 10, 1993, a few days shy of her forty-second birthday, my mother underwent a radical mastectomy of her left breast. The surgery was deemed a "success" by the narrow parameters being used to define the word, given the late stage of her cancer. The new, gigantic tumor was excised along with the breast tissue, but it became clear that the cancer had now moved well beyond her breast and lymph nodes. She spent her last-ever birthday in bed, semi-conscious from the pain medication.

The next stop on my mother's survival tour was a bone marrow transplant clinic in Denver, Colorado. She'd heard of it through a friend of a friend and supposedly the clinic had a promising track record of helping cancer patients into remission by remov-ing their bone marrow, cleaning it out, and injecting it back in. Unlike her previous foray into the world of alternative medicine, this treatment program was legitimate and approved by her medical team.

The protocol would be punishing, including more chemo, and would bring her to the brink of death before it could offer the faintest hope of extending her life. Friends generously covered the air fare and through the close-knit, supportive network of the nationwide Jewish community, my mom stayed with a religious family who kept kosher and were happy to have her for the duration of her treatment. Two and a half weeks after her mastectomy, she and her friend Elaine boarded a plane to Denver, full of hope that she'd return cancer free.

While she was away, my siblings and I tried to cheer her up with telephone calls and home videos of Rivky and Miryam coaxing two-year-old Gita to "sing a song for Mommy," to quote lines from the movie *Aladdin* in her doll-like voice, and of all four sisters in the kitchen making French toast. One video featured our dad self-consciously looking directly into the camera while he told our mom about a bar mitzvah he'd attended. My brother Eli made a brief and rare appearance to use the wall phone in our kitchen before disappearing downstairs to his room while telling the camera that his car window had been broken the night before. My personal favorite: Miryam filming me in my bedroom while I got ready for yet another dreaded blind date to pick me up and I rolled my eyes while cracking sarcastic comments about how "delighted" I was at the prospect. I'd been set up a few times before, never with anyone who made me laugh (the main criteria I gave to the matchmaker) or had anything interesting to say. The bachelors started to merge into a monolith and I'd yet to agree to a second date with any of them. "You're being too picky," the matchmaker said after I'd rejected yet another one of her offerings. The message was clear. I had a bankrupt father and a dying mother, which made me a less-than-sought-after commodity in her world. I was expected to take what I could get and be grateful for it. For no other reason than to appease my mother while she was still alive, I endured the indignities of blind dating.

On this occasion, the guy was a twenty-one-year-old accounting student at Brooklyn College named Avi. There had been zero chemistry during our introductory phone call, but we arranged a time for him to pick me up from home, where I'd been for the weekend, to take me back to my dorm. "Maybe there'll be chemistry when you meet in person" is what the matchmaker (and my mother) said. *If the date is a disaster, at least I'll get a free ride back to the city,* I consoled myself. Miryam and Rivky giggled as we stood by the living room window, watching Avi pull up in his sensible light blue Honda Civic. "Oh, he looks *really cool,* Gi!" Miryam teased as a skinny boy wearing a button-down shirt tucked into chinos walked up our front path. I took note of how similar his outfit was to the one my dad was wearing. "Shut up, Mir," I growled before racing to meet Avi at the door; I didn't want him to come inside. He took my weekend duffel bag and stowed it in the car trunk, then opened the passenger door for me while commenting on alternate routes he might take to Manhattan to avoid traffic. It felt like I was going on a date with my father. After a pasta dinner at a kosher café near my dorm, he dropped me off and said he'd had a nice time. I was already dreading the call I'd make to my mother later to tell her there'd been even less chemistry in person.

It was mid-November when my mother finally came home, physically destroyed but buoyed emotionally by the report that the bone marrow transplant and chemo had worked. There was, according to her latest scans, no evidence of cancer. It was a miracle; it felt too good to be true.

And it was.

By December, her cancer was once again visible on the scans—and this time it was everywhere. Her lesions had metastasized to the point that they presented on the outside of her body on her breastbone and upper back, gruesome and oozing.

She had more radiation, but it wasn't working.

Our prayers weren't working.

Nothing was working.

On a freezing cold Shabbat morning in February, she crept into my room. I'd been sleeping but heard the door creak open. I kept my eyes closed, pretending to be asleep but could feel her hovering over me, could hear her shallow breath rattling through her mouth. I didn't want to look at her. I wasn't prepared to face whatever it was that she'd come to say.

"Gila?" she tried, tentative and weak.

I didn't move.

"Gi?" I focused on breathing deeply and regularly, like a sleeping person would. I hated myself for doing this, for not sitting up, patting my bedspread, and inviting her to come sit with me. For not giving her comfort. I wanted to be that daughter. I wanted us to have heart-to-heart talks, like some of my friends did with their moms. I intuited that I didn't want to hear what she'd come to say. I didn't want to have to tell her that I believed she'd pull through this because I did not. I am a pragmatist whereas my mother is a dreamer. My bed shifted slightly as she perched herself on its edge. Her soft, high-pitched moans and wet, strangled words told me she was crying. I held back my own tears because people don't cry in their sleep.

"Gila, I want you to promise me something," she said, seemingly to no one. "I want you to promise me you'll make sure Tati gets married again. Miryam, Rivky, and Gita are still kids, they need a mother figure. Tati won't be able to do it alone." Her sobs intensified and my bed shook. Still, I "slept." I knew what she'd come looking for and I wasn't sure I could provide it. I felt like a terrible daughter and silently berated myself. *Comfort her*, my brain commanded.

"I'm so scared, Gi. I am so scared. And I'm sorry," she gargle-whispered, the mucus nearly drowning out her words. Words that finally forced me "awake." Whatever complicated interactions my mother and I had shared, I set them aside. Right now, she needed me to be a less terrible daughter.

"Ma?" I squinted at her, hoping to look like someone emerging from a deep slumber. The floodgates opened and she doubled over, nearly falling off my bed. I sidled up to her, hugging her bony shoulders, and tried to think of something comforting to say. I couldn't. There was no comfort to be had. She was dying and we both knew it.

She started her monologue from the beginning, asking me to personally see to it that my father remarried.

"Ma, don't talk like that. Why are you thinking about such things?" I stopped myself from saying "You'll be fine!" even though I wondered if that's what she wanted to hear. She cried on my shoulder. I cried while staring out my window at the snow-covered branches of our weeping cherry tree, my mother's favorite.

Her condition continued to deteriorate through the winter and into spring. I tried to balance schoolwork, my job as a fashion assistant for a junior label, and supporting my sisters in ways I felt capable. My salary allowed me to treat them to the occasional lunch at a fancy NYC restaurant and small purchases at the newly opened Warner Bros. store on 57th Street. More than what we ate and bought, these outings offered Miryam and Rivky a glimpse at what life could look like if they prioritized their education and financial independence after high school.

On a Friday in early June, my mother spiked a fever that left her disoriented. She was rushed back to Lenox Hill hospital. Elaine spent Shabbat with her there while I stayed home with the rest of my family. I'd already been living at home for a month and found being in such close quarters with my mother unbearable. When I changed the dressings on her lesions, I was overcome by her deathly smell and low, persistent moaning. It filled me with a quiet fury. *It didn't have to be like this*, I thought, *you should have stopped this when you still had the chance.*

On Monday, I went to see her in the hospital and when her small, watery eyes eventually landed on me, her joy was so pure, so childlike. It leveled me.

"Gi!" she said slowly, barely audible. "You came!"

I moved closer and took her brittle hand in mine. I studied her crimson nails, the blue topography of her veins. Committing them to memory.

She wished me a "Good Shabbos," the greeting typically used among Jews throughout the twenty-five hours between sundown Friday and when the stars are visible on Saturday. It was Monday.

"Good Shabbos, Gi, Good Shabbos," she said over and over. I turned to Elaine, with my eyebrows knit in confusion.

"*Nebach*, the cancer has spread to her brain," Elaine explained, using the Yiddish word meaning "pity." That's what we had become, the nebach family. Elaine's eyes were red-rimmed and sad. I thought I should feel something, too; I should have been in pain, grieving, consumed with fiery hot rage that my mother was dying, but all I felt was numb.

I watched the jagged, uneven motion of her bony chest rising and falling and squeezed her hand a little bit tighter.

"Good Shabbos, Ma," I said through a long exhale. "I love you."

Wednesday, June 14, 1994. It was early evening and our house was a flurry of activity. My mother's friends swarmed, whispered, tsk-tsk-tsk-ing. They made plans to send Gita to the loving woman who ran her nursery and one of them volunteered to stay at our house with Rivky, who'd seen my mother a few days earlier and understood what was happening. She was a bright, pensive child and had grown up too fast during the years of my mother's illness. Still, she was only ten years old, and we wanted to shield her from the grim scene that awaited us. The rest of us headed to the hospital where my mom had been admitted for nearly a week. We went because my father called from there and said, "You need to come here. Now."

One of my mother's friends kept asking me if I understood what was happening. I wanted to tell her that I'd known what was happening since that day at the airport two years ago, that I felt like I was the only one who'd seen this coming, but I was too tired to be belligerent and simply said, "Yes." Someone drove me and my sister over the Verrazano and through the Lincoln Tunnel to sit and wait for the inevitable.

My uncle—my mother's only sibling—had landed from Israel that morning and brought my grandfather from his home in Brooklyn to say goodbye to his daughter. We all took to our corners of the waiting room, and I could barely stand to look at my uncle as he held his slouched father close. I tried unsuccessfully to banish images of the last time either of them sat shiva after losing a loved one. For my grandfather, it would have been twenty years earlier and my mother would have been with him, probably with me as a newborn cradled in her arms.

We were on death watch and it was painful and awkward. Miryam and I were encouraged to spend a few minutes with our mom and say comforting things, despite the fact that she was sedated and on a ventilator.

"She can hear everything you say," the nurses assured us.

As the eldest, I headed in first and asked everyone else in the room for some privacy.

The bed swallowed my mother whole, the bright lights washing out her already pale complexion. The beeping and hissing machines made me nervous but what I found most disturbing was the surgical tape in the shape of an X on the side of her open, slack mouth. It held the ventilator tube in place. It was unbearable. I pulled up a chair and sat beside her in silence for a few moments, composing my thoughts and crying silently.

"Ma," I breathed into her ear, my cheek pressed to hers, "I love you. You don't have to suffer anymore, it's OK. Don't worry about the kids. I promise to look after them. I promise I'll make you proud." I was twenty years old and could not possibly understand what that promise might look like over the years and decades to come, but I knew they were the right words to say. And I meant every single one of them.

My mother's friend Helen once told me that she'd caught her mother's tears in a tissue as she lay dying, that those tears were precious and to be cherished. I remembered her words as thin rivulets began to slide down my mother's cheeks—she really *could* hear me—and I reached for a tissue from her bedside table. I caught the whole continuous stream, and gently folded that tissue into the pocket of my denim skirt. I exited the room, making space for others to say their goodbyes; there wasn't much time.

My friends had tracked down the number of the nurses' station outside my mom's room and kept calling to offer support.

"Not yet," I told them. "But soon."

A code blue alert blared through the hospital paging system and I knew it was for her. Everyone except for my dad had been instructed to wait outside the room for this final stage. We clustered together, hugging, wiping our noses with linty, crushed up

tissues and our sleeves, shaking our heads. A doctor appeared
from behind her door, walked toward us, said, "I'm sorry. She's
gone." We'd been holding our breath for minutes, hours. Then, it
all came out in a collective, guttural wail.

I was allowed to return to her bedside, and she was still exactly
the same as when I whispered my promises to her, only the plastic peg sticking out of her mouth was no longer connected to a
breathing tube. She was still. Peaceful, but for the peg. It was
disconcerting, an item that had use only minutes before, now use-
less. I wanted to yank it out. I kissed her once on her still-warm,
papery cheek and forced myself to conjure an image of her doing
yoga in the living room, singing "Happy Birthday" while walking
into my bedroom with a double-layered chocolate cake, lighting
the Shabbat candles in her emerald-green velour caftan, mental
snapshots from a time before any of this started. I was now a
motherless daughter, just like her.

2

great at a shiva

The house was teeming with people when we came home from the hospital late that night. We were like industrious ants moving about in a glass terrarium. When we'd last stood in our high-ceilinged living room, it was filled with natural light. Now, it was dark outside and the recessed ceiling bulbs blazed, jarring and unnatural. June 14, the last day my mother had been alive, was about to give way to June 15, the first day of the rest of our motherless lives.

The silent car ride from Manhattan to Staten Island had done little to clear my head and I wasn't ready for the onslaught of well-meaning friends and neighbors. My uncle had driven my grandfather home to Brooklyn for a night of rest before making the trip to Staten Island the next day to bury his eldest child. I was relieved to have a brief respite from bearing witness to their pain. There'd be plenty of that in the week to come as we all sat shiva.

I could already hear footsteps overhead as my father pulled the car into the garage and turned off the engine. In our absence, my parents' friends made quick and thorough work of preparing the house for the grueling week that lay ahead for the mourners. That's what we were now: me, my father, brother, sisters, uncle, and grandfather. Mourners.

"Who the hell turned on the air?" were my father's first words as we opened the metal door between the warm, stuffy garage and the downstairs landing. "It's only June, it was off when we left. What, do I work for the power company?" he fumed half-heartedly.

"Ta, not now," I mumbled. "We can turn it off later, OK?"

"Mamaleh, have you seen our electric bills? They're killing me."

I could say his irritation over the air-conditioning was displaced grief, but the reality was that such concerns were typical for my father. Money was tight and, unlike my mother's exorbitant medical bills, electricity usage could be reined in.

We trudged up the gray carpeted stairs, past the pale pink and gray handrails that used to be wood until my mom had them painted as part of her years-long quest to achieve the silver and pink living room of her dreams. She didn't get very far. The lone piece of furniture in the otherwise empty, high-ceilinged room was a silver upholstered couch she'd custom-ordered. Shortly after its arrival, she gave birth to Gita and then got sick; furnishing the room dropped down the priority list. She couldn't have imagined that the couch she loved so much would be occupied nearly around the clock by people who missed her terribly. The house was being transformed into a place of mourning for the seven days following her funeral: a Shiva House.

The crowd milled quietly around my father who looked pale and out of his depth. They spoke with authority, coaxing him into making a thousand tiny decisions about where to hold the eulogy portion of the proceedings and about the burial, which would take place in United Hebrew Cemetery on Staten Island. I stayed on the other side of the living room, still trying to reconcile how I was feeling (numb, detached, relieved) with how I thought I was supposed to be feeling (devastated, mournful, orphaned). A few women hurried over to me. I asked where Rivky was and was relieved to learn that she'd long since gone to sleep for the night.

"Gila, she loved you so much, your mother," said one of my mom's friends, her face contorted in its own grief.

"Oy, nebach, how she suffered. Thank God she had you kids, you were her pride and joy," said another.

"How she would have loved to have seen you married and danced at your wedding," said one of a handful of people who over the course of the week would make other such well-intended yet unhelpful comments.

"You're like the mother now," one of her friends said through tears, the word "mother" getting caught in her throat as she hugged me close. But I did not want to be the mother, the mama-leh. I wanted to keep my promise to my mother and be the best older sister I could be. I didn't want to stop my life, the one I'd been building dollar by earned dollar on my path to independence. My siblings had lost their mother, but so had I.

I needed space, needed to breathe. Eli and Miryam had snuck off to their rooms. I suddenly felt half my age and escaped to the hallway bathroom where I stood facing the same mirror I'd stood before only hours earlier, wiping my tears and washing my face before leaving for the hospital. But now, instead of seeing my reflection, all I saw was the green and yellow floral-print pillow-case someone had used to cover the mirror, a reminder that during shiva, we were not to concern ourselves with our appearance.

In Judaism, mourning an immediate family member comes with its own detailed list of laws, rituals, and customs. The practices are as much about easing the suffering of the survivors as they are about honoring the deceased. They build an immediate enclosure of support around the aggrieved and continue for one year, allowing for a gentle, gradual reentry into society.

Scenes of a Jewish house of mourning on television or in the movies often feature a huge table laden with a buffet of bagels, cream cheese, and lox, with visitors milling about with small plates of food in their hands. The immediate family, the mourners, alternate between sitting in groups on a sofa, engaging in quiet conversation with the visitors in various parts of the house, and going out for a walk or to run an errand. They are well-dressed and groomed as if they'd just returned from a standard Shabbat service in synagogue. My experience with sitting shiva bears little resemblance to any of this.

My mother's burial would take place the next morning, less than twenty-four hours after she died. In Judaism, it's a sign of respect to the deceased to lay them to rest as quickly as possible and in the interim period between death and the funeral, my family and I would assume the status of onens. This meant we were not permitted to perform any mitzvot as we would under normal circumstances. No praying, no putting on tefillin, no reciting of blessings—all rituals that connect us to God and give structure and meaning to our days. Preparing to bury a family member is so important that it takes precedence over God.

Before going to sleep that night, I showered and washed my hair, letting my natural curls air dry. In accordance with the laws of shiva, I wouldn't be able to shower again until Friday (an exception to the no-washing-for-seven-days rule is preparation for Shabbat) and laid out my funeral outfit: a white button-down blouse and a long black skirt, modest even while sitting low to the ground. The next day, after the eulogy, someone would slice into the collar of my blouse with a razor blade so I could perform the mitzvah of kriya (tearing my garment), which signifies the beginning of the mourning period. I made sure to select a blouse I wouldn't especially miss when it was thrown out after the week's wear, but one that was still clean and ironed. I could hear my mother in my head saying, "Make sure you look nice, you're still on the market and you never know who'll stop by to pay a shiva call."

It was a hot summer's night and my father had mercifully left the air running. As I burrowed deep into my bed, pulling the comforter over my head in an effort to create a sort of sensory deprivation chamber, I heard my bedroom door open followed by footsteps on the hardwood floor. I lowered the blanket just enough to peek out with one eye.

"Gi, can I sleep in your room tonight?" Miryam asked, holding her blanket and pillow.

"Sure, it'll be like a slumber party!" I said with forced gaiety, pulling out the high riser from under my bed. I released the latch, allowing the metal frame to pop up.

Miryam was the quintessential middle child. My parents had nicknamed her "the smiley baby" because of her tendency to always smile, and her determination to make everyone around her happy, too. A natural empath and nurturer, fourteen-year-old Miryam found that she was in need of some tenderness herself. She was at the very end of her freshman year in high school, a challenging time in a teenager's life under even the best circumstances. Now, on top of that, she also had to navigate this terrible new terrain. It was my turn to play the role of nurturer for Miryam.

We'd been taught to recite the Shema prayer at bedtime as soon as we could talk and tonight we whispered it together. Considered the most essential of all Jewish prayers, it declares

God's singularity and kingship, and its recitation is also a request for God's protection. The same prayer appeared on the scrolls inside mezuzahs that hung on every doorpost in our home. As onens, Miryam and I were technically forbidden from saying the Shema as we were still in that limbo state between death and mourning, but I didn't mention that to her. That night we said the words not out of obligation, but out of comfort. If it was the worst transgression I ever committed against my faith, I could live with that.

"Did anyone tell Rivky yet?" she wondered as we lay facing each other, bone tired yet wide awake.

"I'm not sure, Mir," I yawned, half hoping that someone else had broken the news to her. "Let's get some sleep and we'll deal with it in the morning. Tomorrow is a big day."

"OK, but promise me you'll make sure Rivky knows. I don't want to be the one to have to tell her," she mumbled, finally drifting off to sleep.

"I promise. Love you." It was a relief that we had to tell only one of our sisters; Gita, three years old and already accustomed to living in a house without a mother, wouldn't know the difference. The downside of this, of course, was that Gita would likely have very few memories of her.

Early the next morning, I left Miryam in bed and steeled myself before entering Rivky's bedroom. I sat on the edge of her bed, watching the comforter rise and fall with her breath and feeling sick to my stomach. "Rivky, Pivky . . ." I stroked her silky red hair, coaxing her out of what I hoped had been a sweet dream. She sat up, forcing me to look into her sad brown eyes. "Um, so we went to see Mommy last night in the hospital and, uh, and she's gone to a better place." I grimaced at myself for relying on such a clichéd choice of words, but I'd come unprepared. "Do you understand what I'm saying? She won't have to suffer anymore," I said, unable to bear the sight of her anguished face and drawing her close for a hug. My little sister sobbed into my shoulder and her skinny body shook. She understood.

Later that morning, Miryam and I sat in the kitchen, picking at some Entenmann's cookies for breakfast. It felt wrong on two levels.

1. We were in the habit of making a blessing on food before consuming it but as onens could not do so.

2. My mother would not have approved of cookies for breakfast. A health-food nut, she barely allowed them, or any other junk food, to be eaten no matter what time of day it was.

I abandoned my unhealthy breakfast and went to find my father by the glass porch door overlooking the street we'd lived on for nearly twenty years. I'd seen him wrap his tefillin around his arm and drape himself in a tallis in that very spot more times than I could count. Now he just stood there in a dark blazer and white shirt, gently shaking his head while holding his mug of instant coffee and staring out the window. No tefillin. No tallis. No wife.

I joined him and together we stared at the same irreverently sunny sky.

"What am I going to do without her, Gi?" he asked, turning to me in despair. "What are we going to do?" He looked truly lost.

"It'll be OK, Ta," I offered, remembering the promise I'd made to my mother less than twenty-four hours earlier. My words were as much for his benefit as for my own. A gray sedan turned the corner at the top of our street and slowed as it neared our house. My father and I watched my uncle park the car and help his father and stepmother, whom we affectionately called Babi Becky (pronounced "Bobby Becky"), carry their bags up our walkway.

"I'll get the door and then wake Eli up," I said, bracing myself. "It's almost time to go."

The eulogy took place in a room lit with fluorescent lights at the Young Israel of Staten Island. It was standing room only and the crowd spilled out onto the streets. Faigie Reinitz was a well-liked woman who'd generously given her time and creativity to the community. Her diminutive frame and impossibly slender wrists and ankles belied her big personality. At only five foot two inches (five foot four inches after a perm at Fickle Fingers, her favorite hair salon), she had a charisma that made people turn whenever she entered a room. She smiled with her eyes and put anyone she encountered immediately at ease. People from her past and present came out in droves to pay their respects.

As in the Orthodox Jewish tradition, men and women were seated separately with an aisle down the middle. Miryam, Rivky, Babi Becky, and I sat up front, shoulder to shoulder on the varnished wooden pew, a few feet away from my father, uncle, grandfather, and Eli. Gita remained with her nursery caretaker. A funeral was no place for a three-year-old.

On his way to the wooden lectern before us, the rabbi crouched down next to me and asked if I'd like to say a few words. I did, more than a few words in fact. I wanted to tell the assembled masses about my creative mother who'd always made our Purim costumes by hand, whose skill with a staple gun, needle and thread, and tailors' shears were nothing short of surgical, to publicly acknowledge her for influencing my own creative inclinations. I wanted to say that thanks to the reminders she'd hammered into me to call my grandparents every Friday they were now a permanent part of my routine and how sad I was that my future children wouldn't be able to call her. I wanted to say that when I was little, I thought she was the most exquisitely beautiful woman in existence. I wanted to share that I knew about the secret stash of Kit Kats she kept in her bedside-table drawer and how, although she must have known that I, her chocolate-loving daughter, was the one covertly reducing the inventory, she'd replenish her (our) supply without ever confronting me.

But I said none of these things. I was too overwhelmed, too self-conscious of being an object of pity, too terrified of the communal expectation that I pause my life to pick up where my mother left off, so I shook my head and looked away. The rabbi did not press me further.

My mother's coffin, a simple pine box draped in a tallis, was carried in by several men and placed on a pedestal between my family and the rabbi. I couldn't tell you what he spoke about. Mentally, I was one week into the future when the madness of the funeral and shiva would dissipate, and was wondering what life would look like, and if it would be any different from how it had already been for months. I kept thinking that life would be easier without the constant waiting for scan results, the relentless medical bills that kept my father up at night, the never-ending refrain of "How's your mom doing?" from family and friends. I swatted away the thought, knowing it was terrible, but it kept popping up, like a game of Whac-A-Mole where, instead of moles, there was guilt.

My father, whose slight build, enormous eyes, and thick, wavy hair had always given him a youthful appearance, today looked a decade older than his forty-four years as he struggled through tears to adequately convey to the congregation how highly he thought of his wife, how much he'd miss her. My grandfather wore a confused yet resigned expression, like he was trying to make sense of the fact that despite having survived the concentration camps, a death march, moving to a foreign country nearly

penniless, the death of his wife—herself a Holocaust survivor—
at forty-nine, here he sat staring at a box containing his only
daughter. He repeatedly dabbed his red-rimmed eyes and leaky
nose with his cloth handkerchief, not bothering to return it to his
breast pocket as he normally would.

"The burial will take place at Hebrew National Cemetery," the
rabbi's voice boomed, snapping me back to the present as two of
my parents' friends approached the front pews with razor blades
in their shaking hands. My father's closest friend Irwin was tasked
with slicing the garments of my father, brother, uncle, and grandfather while Elaine did the same for me and my sisters. Each of us
grabbed hold of our sliced collars and yanked. The quietly violent
sound of ripping cotton and wool was like a starting gun, signaling
the commencement of our mourning. Whatever trance I'd been in
was broken by the *kkrrrrrrrr* of my collar being torn close to my
ear. The shift in my status was palpable.

Although Babi Becky was the only grandmother we'd ever
known, having married our grandfather when I was only five,
she was not a blood relative and therefore not a mourner in the
eyes of the Jewish law. She sat with us during the services and
was regarded by all in attendance as if she'd lost a daughter, but
she did not tear her clothes and would spend the coming week as
one of the swarm of people who'd serve our meals and tidy up
rather than sit shiva alongside us. Out of the corner of my eye, I
saw her watching us tearing kriya, the gnarled, arthritic fingers of
one hand clamped tightly over her mouth as she shook her head
and squeezed tears out of rheumy eyes behind her coke-bottle
glasses. Her exclusion from the ritual felt unfair. I made a point of
hugging her just then, softly saying, "I'm sorry, Babi, I'm sorry,"
while she sobbed on my shoulder, the smell of mothballs and
talcum powder amplifying the nausea I'd been keeping at bay all
morning.

The congregation remained standing as the coffin was carried back down the aisle and out into the bright June sunshine to a waiting hearse. My family and I followed, passing through a blur of sad faces and murmured condolences as we were escorted to the cars that would take us on the short drive to the cemetery. Rivky was whisked away to her friend's house.

I sat in the back of a sedan with Eli and Miryam while a family friend drove in a long, slow procession. To his credit, he didn't try to make conversation. If he overheard our less than mournful chatter, he gave no indication.

Me: *deep, audible sigh* This is just crazy.

Miryam: Yeah.

Eli: Guys, you know the cemetery is on a street called Arthur Kill Road, right? Arthur *Kill*, get it?

That got a half chuckle/half groan out of me and my sister, which then morphed into giggles before ballooning into maniacal laughter, bringing more tears to our already puffy, red eyes.

We retreated into the silence of our own minds for a few minutes, staring out the windows at the cars full of people on their way to do things other than bury their mothers. The car slowed as it made its way down a hill and a large sign that read "United Hebrew Cemetery" came into view. The driver cleared his throat and said, "We're almost there, OK?" while eyeing us in the rearview mirror and noting that, all things considered, we were, in fact, OK.

At the bottom of the hill and just outside the entrance of the cemetery was a small, old-timey pub bearing a sign advertising its offerings which, in an Old English font, read "Fine Food and Spirits." Our eyes landed on the word "spirits" and we looked at one another wondering who was going to say it first. I stepped up to the plate:

Me: Guys, fine food and *spirits*!

We absolutely lost it. It was the last time we laughed that day. Regaining our composure as we piled out of the car, we followed the funeral director and immediately sobered upon seeing the pallbearers carefully maneuvering my mother's casket on slats above a freshly dug grave. My father, uncle, grandfather, and Babi were already there as throngs of people made their way toward us.

Usually, at a Jewish funeral, the crowd at a burial site is much smaller than the one at the eulogy. But nothing about this was usual. This was an abject tragedy, and many people were reluctant to leave us until we had the sort of closure that only a burial could offer. My family and I stood as close as possible to the mouth of the grave. Surrounding us were layers and layers of people, as far as the eye could see. My friends Chani, Suri, and Tamar inched their way through the crowd and positioned themselves by my side. A low, fizzing current was running through me on a loop, and I felt cold sweat begin to pool under my armpits. I was grateful to have my friends surrounding me like sentient guards, ready to catch me if I fell, in any sense of the word.

The rabbi chanted a prayer called *El Maleh Rachamim*, recognizing God's compassion, and praying for my mother's soul. He nodded in my father's direction, signaling that it was time. The casket was slowly lowered into the ground to the sounds of big, gulping sobs and high-pitched wails from anyone with a view over and through the crowds. The lethal combination of heat and grief, and a realization that I'd never have an adult relationship with my mother, never have the chance to rectify those past few turbulent teenage years, knocked the wind out of me and I slumped forward. Tamar and Chani caught me under my (extremely wet) armpits just before I hit the ground.

My father, uncle, and brother each took turns digging a shovelful of dirt then scattering it over the casket. The rest of the men present stepped forward one by one, shoveling, scattering, and passing to the next in line. Although it is customary for men to participate in this final portion of a burial, I have no doubt that had I asked, the shovel would have quickly been passed to me, but I had neither the emotional nor physical strength required for the job. My grandfather's head shook gently while he said over and over, "This is not in nature," meaning it was not the natural order of things to bury a child. Still, he dug the rusting, iron shovel into the pile of dirt and lay its contents on the coffin. This man who'd already suffered enough for ten men in his lifetime, who maybe thought he'd survived the worst life could sling at him, was now burying his daughter.

We turned and the crowds split in half like a flash mob performing a well-rehearsed choreography. We walked through them and back to our cars, back to our new lives as the family without a mother.

The definitive guide to the rituals of shiva is a book called *The Jewish Way in Death and Mourning* by Rabbi Maurice Lamm. Several copies awaited my family upon our return from the cemetery, dropped off by our shul. The books were part of a bigger tableau that included special mourner chairs that were low to the ground, a folding table covered in twenty-four-hour yahrzeit candles, a portable aron kodesh (an ark) containing a small torah scroll for daily morning prayers, and a stack of well-worn siddurim, or prayer books.

In most shiva houses, mourners sit together in one spacious area, usually the living room. But we were too many people, of too many ages, with too many friends. So, aside from that first day of shiva when we banded together to try to mourn as a team, my siblings and I scattered around the house and sat in our own little clusters.

After wordlessly picking at a meal that included the requisite hardboiled eggs—a symbol of the circle of life—we took our places sitting in the semicircle of short-legged mourning chairs. A handful of close friends who'd escorted us from the burial sat facing us in seats of a normal height and were the first to officially offer their condolences. They were performing the mitzvah of being *menachem avel*, the term used for a condolence call which means "comforting the mourners" and over the course of the week, it would be standing room only for most of our waking hours. Being menachem avel ranks pretty highly as mitzvot go and it's not unusual for community members with even the loosest ties to the deceased to visit a shiva house.

Comforting a mourner is not easy. Sitting with someone else's pain can be deeply uncomfortable. While the week of shiva is an opportunity to remember the deceased, it's really about comforting the mourners in their time of grief while they forgo creature comforts like freshly laundered clothes and listening to music. It's harder to offer comfort to someone when what they are allowed to receive is so limited (although there was no limit to how much food we could have). Seeing the forlorn faces of my mother's friends, hearing them reminisce about how she was the life of the party and loved to laugh didn't bring me comfort so much as it amplified the tragedy of her death. "You should know no more tsuris"—may no more hardship befall you—was the typical refrain by visitors who tried to wish us well in the face of such devastation. I found this protocol less comforting, more overwhelming.

For me, comfort meant sitting with my friends, tucked away downstairs in my room. It meant being a twenty-year-old with other twenty-year-olds who understood what I needed most: to alleviate the heaviness of the atmosphere with laughter. Besides, my mother had been so sick for so long, my grief over her death was balanced by relief that her suffering was finally over.

I dragged my shiva chair downstairs and held court there. My siblings and I retreated to our corners to grieve privately because watching each other do it was too unbearable, mirroring back on ourselves what we looked like. Gita, with her blue eyes, flaming red curls, and pillowy cheeks brought all of us the most comfort. She flitted from room to room, sometimes sitting on my father's lap, sometimes tearing through my room and squealing with laughter while my friends chased her, bringing joy to mourners and visitors alike with her blissful ignorance. Her presence, of course, highlighted the sheer magnitude of our loss.

Early the next morning, several men arrived to form a minyan, the group of ten men required for Shacharit, thus kicking off the first full day of shiva. Miryam, Rivky, and I would have been welcome to join the services from the adjacent dining room or kitchen but did not count toward a minyan and, frankly, we were just as happy to sleep a bit later before the waves of visitors began to arrive.

Neighbors got to work triaging the parade of food that flowed in. Pans of lasagna, a large platter of deli meat, cookies, chocolate babka cakes, meatballs and spaghetti . . . All this was before the days of those handy meal-planner websites. My family held by the rule that food brought into a shiva house did not leave. So, it was either consumed by us, a bunch of sad people whose movement was limited and were therefore not building up much of an appetite, or it was disposed of. Some of it was frozen to be eaten sometime later that week/month/year/decade. Tamar, by far the most organized of my friends, made herself busy rearranging pans and containers of food in both the kitchen freezer and the spare one in the basement like some culinary game of Tetris, until there was simply no more space. One time, Babi Becky caught her doing this and went ballistic that she was wasting food even though the stuff Tamar got rid of was inedible. Thirty years later, when I asked Tamar what she remembered most about my mother's shiva, it was this encounter with Babi Becky.

The Jewish Way in Death and Mourning is full of guidelines on how to mourn, but that didn't stop some people from adding their own made-up rules. Sometimes (often) my friends comforted me a little too well and our cackling carried up to the living room overhead where the mood was considerably more somber. Once, when our decibel level reached unreasonable heights, our neighbor Magda cracked open my bedroom door, poked her head in, and hissed in her thick Hungarian accent, "Excuse me ladies, please, this is very inappropriate," before turning to me with "Gila, you're sitting shiva, come on!" as if I'd for one second thought there might be another explanation as to why I was sitting on my childhood bedroom floor in a ripped shirt with greasy hair, surrounded by my friends who'd driven in from Brooklyn, Englewood, and Silver Spring, Maryland, among other places, in the middle of a Monday morning in June.

"Sorry," I mumbled, meeting her judgmental gaze while keeping my head tilted down. But I wasn't sorry. This was *my* shiva, *my* mother who had died, *my* place to say how I'd mourn—and laughter, last time I'd checked, wasn't on the "don't" list of the book. But I was too tired to tell her any of this and I let it go. Until she left the room, that is. We counted to ten and exploded into more laughter.

Among my visitors was Max who'd just graduated from Yeshiva University with a degree in finance and had recently joined the list of guys I'd been set up with. What distinguished Max from my previous, ill-fated blind dates was his wry sense of humor and our mutual love of reading. He had an advantage in that a friend rather than the matchmaker had introduced us. We'd met two months earlier and, by the time my mother died, had been out to dinner, the movies, and walks in Central Park close to a dozen times. Was I attracted to Max? Not especially. But he was compassionate and thoughtful and answered my insomniac phone calls in the middle of the night during my time of grief. I appreciated his attention. My mother never met him but had been hopeful about our prospects; after all, he was a nice YU boy from a fancy neighborhood. When I broke up with Max a few weeks after shiva, he asked me to consider him a friend and to call if I ever needed anything.

On day three of shiva, Max brought a huge deli platter (such a mensch) for lunch. A man I didn't recognize intercepted my family's attempts to dig in. "No meat allowed," he insisted, snapping the clear, circular lid back onto the enormous plastic base.

"Are you sure?" I challenged. "I don't think that's right."

"Eating meat is a sign of celebration; of course you can't have meat," he said confidently, but after consulting some other adults present and noting that we'd been eating roast chicken and meatballs for dinner all week, we double checked The Book. He was wrong. Sitting shiva was hard enough, we didn't need any extra made-up rules to further our suffering.

Some of the legitimate rules were overbearing, and I took to finding loopholes around them. For instance, mourners are not allowed to wear laundered clothes and that includes underwear. Remember, we weren't showering either, so you do the math. I reasoned that if someone else wore my underwear for a couple of hours, they'd no longer be considered "laundered" so Suri and Chani took several pairs of my cotton briefs and wore them *over their own*, thank you very much, and that is all you need to know about my creative problem-solving skills.

The week went on this way until it almost felt normal.

The start of each day was signaled by the tinkling of my father's spoon against a glass mug as he stirred his Taster's Choice instant coffee, followed by men's footsteps coming up the stairs, and then Shacharit—morning prayers ending with the Mourner's Kaddish recited by my father, brother, uncle, and grandfather.

Miryam, Rivky, and I would emerge from our bedrooms ready to receive the day's endless stream of visitors. The wafting smell of tuna salad, toasted challah, blintzes, or pasta meant that someone would soon be asking if any of us wanted to take a short break to eat lunch in the kitchen. We didn't always want to. It was awkward to excuse ourselves when expectant visitors were standing right in front of us.

Another influx of men in the evening told us that it was time for Mincha and Maariv, the evening and night-time prayers followed by more recitations of Kaddish. At night, the number of visitors ballooned with people coming after work. It was a grueling schedule, but comforting in its predictability and effective in keeping us constantly engaged until nighttime when exhaustion would yank us into sleep before we had time to wallow in our pain. Each visit concluded with someone standing over us while reading the handwritten Hebrew words from a sign taped to the living room wall. The English translation was: "May the Lord comfort you among the mourners of Zion and Jerusalem."

Seven days after burying my mother, it was time to get up from shiva. After the Shacharit prayer, the men dissipated, our rabbi staying behind to usher us into our next phase of mourning.

"In a few moments, we'll step outside and take a walk up the block," he instructed. "It symbolizes your first steps back into the normal rhythm of life and officially marks the beginning of your shloshim period."

On my way out, I paused in front of a familiar photo in the hallway. It's a sepia-toned, old-timey saloon shot taken during the only family vacation we ever took to Disney World. Per the photographer's directions, no one is smiling so we all have an acute case of resting bitch face. My mom used to stand before the portrait and comment on how jowly she looked in the photo—"I look like a chipmunk, Gi!"— touching her fingertips to her face and gently pulling it up and back. She couldn't have been more than thirty-seven at the time. I'd always thought she looked elegant and pretty in that photo. I still did, and now I wondered if, in seventeen years, I'd think I looked like a chipmunk, too.

Losing our mother at the beginning of the summer allowed for a soft landing in terms of figuring out our new normal. My sisters had finished the school year, and I was living at home until the start of the new semester. My mother's close friends continued to drop in with trays of hot food, to check on us, and to perhaps conjure their friend's memory by standing in her house.

"You'll drop out of college now and run the household, right?" was an assumption more than one of them made. Out loud. To my face.

With as much civility as I could muster, I assured them that Miryam and my father would manage while I worked and finished school and that I'd be home to help on the weekends. I resented them for being so cavalier about my future, for placing such little value on my career and education, both of which I saw as a path to the stability my mother lacked. My future also depended on me avoiding breast cancer and I turned my attention to learning how to protect myself. I dug through a stack of her medical records and found her oncologist's phone number. I told the receptionist who I was and why I was calling, and she choked up.

"Your mom was something special, you know, hon? We really miss her around here," she sniffled before giving me the name and contact details for a breast specialist. "You take good care of yourself, OK?" I assured her that was exactly what I planned to do.

By mid-July, our shloshim period, the first thirty days of mourning, came to an end. We began the slow transition back to everyday life by doing normal things that were forbidden during shloshim, such as cutting our hair. My father and Eli shaved their thirty-day-old beards and went to the barber. My sisters and I didn't need haircuts, but my legs and armpits were in dire need of a Gillette razor. A bereaved spouse is required to mourn for only one month after the funeral, so this marked the end of mourning for my dad. My siblings and I, on the other hand, began avey-lut, in which children mourn their parents for one full year out of respect. We'd have to abstain from attending large gatherings and celebrations, which would be especially difficult for me as my friends were starting to get married, but I appreciated how the mourning rituals were structured to gently ease us into normalcy. Only one month of grieving would have felt too abrupt.

In August, my father went on a date, his first since meeting my mother in 1972.

In September, I stuffed my belongings into a few black garbage bags and moved back into my East 34th Street dorm for my senior year.

3

can we skip to the good parts?

The summer felt interminable. When September finally rolled around, we were grateful for the structure it brought with the preparation for school and the Jewish High Holidays. It would be our first Rosh Hashana and Yom Kippur without our mother, and I hoped I'd remember to gently scratch my sisters' backs for comfort during services the way my mom used to do for me. There were a lot of painful firsts during our year of aveylut: navigating the school-supplies section of Kmart for the girls, our first family photo next to the lit Chanukah menorah with six people instead of seven, the first time we considered what to do with her drawers full of clothes and worthless trinkets whose sentimental value we'd never know.

The lasts were just as painful. The last tube of toothpaste our mom had bought, finding a note or camp letter in her often illegible handwriting, Miryam and Rivky outgrowing dresses our mother had bought when she'd been healthy enough to drive to her favorite New Jersey discount stores.

I moved back into my dorm, began my senior year at college, and resumed my job as a marketing assistant at a small fashion company. Miryam started tenth grade, Rivky went off to sixth, and Gita continued in day care. Eli had opted out of higher education and was now a budding entrepreneur living with friends in Queens. September also heralded my father's favorite season: the one when the running of neither heat nor air-conditioning was required. The season lasted as long as my dad said it did, or until the kids threatened to stage a revolt.

From September to May, I juggled a nearly full-time work schedule and five classes per semester, and attended countless weddings. It wasn't uncommon for people in my circles to get married during or just after their senior year of college. In keeping with the "no major social interactions" rule of mourning, I mostly sat in corridors just outside the grand rooms where the receptions were held. Sometimes I'd be assigned a job to do inside the wedding hall that would make my presence there utilitarian rather than celebratory. Either way, it was depressing to feel like an outsider at such joyous events. It bothered me more than I cared to admit that my friends were getting married while I was not. It didn't matter that I was twenty or twenty-one. It didn't matter that I was far from ready. But it felt like the chasm between us—those who had two parents who loved them and were in a position to pay for huge weddings, who worked because they wanted to and not because they had rent and bills to pay—was widening. Still, I could hear my mother's voice telling me to use the weddings as an opportunity to hunt for a husband. She'd have been pleased to see me back at my pre-gap-year dress size and, thanks to the wizardry of makeup artists (compliments of my bridal friends), looking like a contender.

Most of my weekends were still spent on Staten Island, where I tried to be a decent big sister. Miryam had the household impressively under control, even by adult standards; the place was clean and well-stocked with groceries. Piles of clean, folded laundry on the living room couch were a common sight; washed dishes lay drying upside down on the kitchen counters; the bathrooms smelled passably OK. It was Miryam, not me, who had stepped into the role of "little mommy." She was a born nurturer with energy to burn, always at her best when tending to the needs of others. Perhaps this was also how she processed her grief.

My own coping methods included throwing myself into work and school and surrounding myself with people who could stomach my dark jokes about orphanhood. My repertoire included frequent comments about how lucky my future husband would be to not have a mother-in-law. There were a few other students in my college who'd also lost a parent and together we formed an exclusive club. Our most notable achievement was coming up with the club's name, The Dead Parents Society. Membership was open to anyone who met the following criteria.

1. Grieving at least one parent

2. Dark sense of humor

3. Zero interest in pity

We didn't do much other than eat cafeteria snacks in a small airless classroom and swap anecdotes about friends complaining bitterly about their parents before catching themselves in front of us and awkwardly backpedaling their gripes. For some reason, the group photo we took was not featured alongside the Drama, Debate, and Literary Journal clubs in the yearbook.

While I remained buckled into my continued state of mourning, my father was free to move about the cabin, so to speak, and for him, the cabin was the dating pool and he plunged in headfirst. A father of five, widowed, bankrupt, and living in a house skating on the edge of foreclosure, my handsome, forty-five-year-old dad was a catch nonetheless because that's how lopsided the dating scene is. By the time we all went back to school, my father had met Dafna, a twice-divorced Israeli woman who spoke too loudly, had an open-mouthed smile like the Joker, and whose broad-shouldered, imposing frame was out of sync with my slight father's. She was also a good inch taller than him, which meant she was several inches taller than me and my sisters who shared our mother's pint-size build. He was immediately taken with her, likely because she met all of his criteria: Israeli, not unattractive, and interested in him.

My sisters and I disliked her instantly. We knew our dad needed a woman in his life, but this particular woman did not belong in our family. She was neither nurturing nor capable and those were two things my sisters and I needed most. Soon after he brought her home to meet us, she vanished as suddenly as she'd appeared.

"Dafna went to, eh, Israel to visit her family," my father explained, not that we'd asked about her disappearance. We'd simply high-fived each other, thankful she'd saved us the headache of having to convince our father she wasn't the one. "She wants to take things, eh, slowly." It was the first and only thing about her that I appreciated, and I hoped my father would take this page out of her playbook and put the brakes on his hunt for a spouse. He didn't.

By December, he was engaged to a delightful woman named Lonnie, a warm, soft-spoken widow from a fancy part of Long Island. She seemed genuinely interested in getting to know us and didn't seem to mind slumming it in Staten Island. Her kids were all around the same ages as us and, most fascinating to me, she was American. Like *really* American, with American parents who were Jewish yet spoke perfect English without an accent.

For Chanukah, she gave me, Miryam, and Rivky dainty pearl necklaces nestled in gray velvet boxes. I'd never been gifted a real piece of jewelry before, certainly not one that had been purchased especially for me. I knew it was just a matter of time before Lonnie found out that my dad was broke, and his full head of dark hair and encyclopedic knowledge of the rise and fall of the Roman Empire wouldn't be enough to keep her around.

"This won't last," I whispered to Miryam out of the corner of my mouth while she fastened my new necklace around my neck. We were sitting around our dining table laden with latkes, jam-filled donuts, and chocolate gelt, also provided by Lonnie. "She's too good to be true."

"Yeah, I know," she quietly agreed. "Poor Ta, how will he ever find someone? Here, help me with mine," and she turned, lifting her hair, while my father and Lonnie, seated at the opposite end of the table, made goo-goo eyes at each other. "I hope we at least get to keep these after she's gone," Miryam whispered, touching her necklace and echoing my own thoughts.

A week later, Lonnie returned the two-carat diamond engagement ring my father had given her—the one he'd inherited when his mother passed away years earlier—and asked her now ex-fiancé to extend her deepest apologies to his kids that things didn't work out. At least, that's what my father told us she said.

In February, not long after this inevitable yet disappointing loss, my father brought home another American woman, Carrie, who was in her early thirties and closer in age to me than to my father. She was divorced with a four-year-old daughter and complained often and loudly in her duck honk of a voice. We begged our dad not to marry her, but he proposed again with his mother's ring. This engagement was even shorter than the previous one and the ring was back in its box on his nightstand within a week.

I turned twenty-one on a cold January day, somewhere between Engagements 1 and 2. Contrary to what I'd seen in the movies, there was no car with an oversize bow in the driveway, no all-night bar hopping, no fanfare to celebrate becoming an adult. Instead, I did the most adult thing I could think of, which was to take Miryam and Rivky on a day out it the city. We got dressed up (in photos of that day I'm wearing a black wool beret and a full face of makeup; Miryam, fifteen, is wearing a black swing coat, sunglasses, and my mother's vintage platform shoes), and we went to the Guggenheim Museum (*très* sophisticated!), the Warner Bros. store where we played around with Marvin the Martian dolls, imitating his anodyne voice, and dinner at My Most Favorite Dessert, a kosher pasta and fish restaurant where my sisters and I clinked *L'Chaim* with Coke-filled wine glasses.

My roommates surprised me with a cake and a single can of Coors Light in our dorm room and old friends at other universities called to wish me a "Happy Twenty-First" on my dorm phone. The beer was a gag gift; I'd never had a drink in my life and my only exposure to beer had been when my dad drank it out of an oversize crystal goblet during Shabbat lunch each Saturday. Even from across the table, I thought it smelled like sweaty feet and couldn't imagine that it would taste like anything else. It turned out I was right.

A full month had passed since Carrie had come and gone and no new potential stepmoms had materialized. Perhaps my father was regrouping, being more selective about the women he agreed to meet.

And then.

I was home one weekend in March, and halfway through Friday night dinner, my father casually mentioned that he'd soon be off to Israel for a week. He said he had business there.

"Oh yeah?" I eyed him suspiciously while dunking a hunk of challah into my bowl of chicken matzo ball soup from Kosher Island takeout. "What kind of 'business'?"

Miryam and Rivky stopped slurping and looked at him, their silver spoons hovering over gold-edged bowls, my mother's wedding china. Gita, now four years old, was oblivious as she giggled and hid under the glass table.

"I have business, OK? Some people I have to meet, potential opportunities to, eh, import some table linens and other things."

For as long as I could remember, my father was in the home goods manufacturing and sales business. He had an entrepreneurial spirit and that, combined with an MBA and my mother's encouragement to leave his stable finance job and pursue his American dream, convinced him that being his own boss was the best path to success. Whether it was bad luck, bad business or both, he struggled to gain a solid foothold with any of his companies and when one went bust, he'd file Chapter 11 and start another, often naming the companies after our family. As a little kid, I'd accompany my dad to his midtown Manhattan showroom, which was filled with hanging wall racks and small display tables covered in the linens he manufactured; floral prints, cotton waffle weaves, white-on-white jacquard and, the fabric he was most proud of, Visa by Dacron. It was a brand-new stain-releasing fabric that was made, as the huge American flag on the label indicated, in the USA. That meant something to my immigrant father, supporting the economy of his adoptive country. I'd feel giddy with pride whenever I saw the gold-lettered plaque outside the showroom door bearing the company name: Gila International, Inc. The company folded within a couple of years, but I was secretly smug about being the only one of my siblings to have a business named after me.

My father was still in the home goods business, but now worked out of the basement of his childhood home in Borough Park, Brooklyn. The rest of the house was occupied by rent-paying tenants who'd moved in shortly after my grandfather passed away. As for having "business in Israel," there had been a time in the mid-eighties when he imported home décor from a Tel Aviv–based manufacturer. As much as he loved America, his heart was in Israel, so doing business there was an excuse for frequent visits. It was years since he'd last worked with an Israeli exporter.

I called him out on his "business trip" announcement. "Ta, you don't have business in Israel, why are you really going?" I pressed, salting my already too salty soup and motioning to my sisters to eat up so we could move on to the next course.

"Yes, I do. I can't give you details right now. And anyway, I want to visit Zaidy's *kever*. It's been a while and I miss him," he countered, referring to his father's grave on a mountaintop outside Jerusalem. My dad had decided to bury him there and spoke of someday moving his mother's remains from a cemetery in Brooklyn. This never happened.

"If you say so," I said, already on my way to the kitchen to get the lemon chicken Miryam had prepared and the three kugels—potato, sweet noodle, and broccoli—that my dad had bought that morning.

He went to Israel a few days later, and upon his return, called a family meeting, even summoning my brother home. He had great news to share. "Well, you'll never guess who I ran into at the Kotel," he beamed. "Dafna! Can you believe it?"

We could not.

"Last time I checked, the Kotel has a pretty solid dividing wall between the men's and women's sections, Ta," I pointed out. "How'd you 'run into her' there?" Miryam looked nervous. Rivky looked confused. Eli looked like he was already mentally back in Queens.

"Come on, Gi, you know what I mean, we met on the plaza," he said impatiently, referring to the plaza immediately in front of the Western Wall where it is not uncommon for Jews to run into people from their pasts. "Anyway, we got to talking and went to dinner and it, uh, things are pretty serious between us. We're going to get engaged soon." He proposed the following week. And that was that. Dafna won the game of We Pass the Ring Around.

To her credit, Dafna insisted that the wedding be delayed until after our year of mourning, but in the run-up, she was a constant and invasive presence. Miryam and Rivky were annoyed; they had the house running just fine and didn't want any interference, much less from an overbearing woman who would sing in the bathroom lest anyone hear the sound of her urinating.

While in his dating era, my father would make dramatic proclamations about his children needing a mother. My sisters, who'd be standing right there while my father spoke past them, would desperately protest, "No, we don't, Ta! We're doing fine!" The truth was, he was lonely and had been during the years my mother was sick.

In Dafna, he had an around-the-clock set of ears ready to listen to him discuss (deliver a soliloquy on) Middle Eastern politics, the dangerously low level of water in the Kinneret in Israel, the contributions of John Maynard Keynes to modern-day economics, and conspiracy theories about the cure for cancer already existing but being blocked by Big Pharma for their own financial gain. If Dafna was able to follow what he was saying, it wasn't readily apparent in her frozen smile, rapid blinking, or from her habit of snapping her fingers as she hummed, the two rhythms completely out of sync. She became an annoying fixture in our household, and there was nothing my sisters and I could do about it.

That May, I graduated with a Bachelor of Arts in English Literature and an associate's degree in Judaic Studies. The ceremony took place at Madison Square Garden and as I walked down the aisle with my friends and fellow graduates in our black caps and gowns, I spotted my father, brother, and sisters in the crowd, cheering me on. I blinked back tears and tried not to think of how proud my mom would have been to see me, the first person on her side of the family to reach this milestone. I also tried to block out the sight of Dafna, red lipstick smeared from her attempts at a two-fingered wolf whistle, who I had foolishly hoped would have known better than to come.

The following month marked a year since my mother died. My father, siblings, and I gathered around her grave to bring our mourning to an official close. A handful of close friends were present, too. Dafna had the decency to stay away. In a ceremony called an unveiling, a cloth was pulled away from the newly erected tombstone that we were all seeing for the first time. Seeing her name with her birth and death dates was surreal and I understood why it was customary to wait a year before facing the harsh permanence of a final grave marker. Our rabbi said a few words about how much her absence was felt. My dad then rested one hand on the stone and spoke about life moving on (for some more quickly than others) and how proud she would have been of her kids. Through tears, I studied the English and Hebrew words engraved on the stone: her name, Faiga Leah bat Natan, and dates of her birth and death. The rest of the text was a tribute I'd written, at my father's request. I struggled to find the perfect words to convey to future visitors who and what she was. What do you write about your mom when you're twenty-one that will still hold weight when you're forty? Or fifty or sixty if you're blessed enough to outlive her?

I wrote about her pursuit of truth and justice, her modesty, her unwavering support of her husband, and finished with the Hebrew words for this sentiment: "There is not enough space on this stone to list all of her good deeds."

My eyes continued to scan the tombstone, to take in this blunt reality, and a growing sense of unease crept through me. Something felt off. I read it from top to bottom once more and groaned. "Hey," I said, turning to my friend Chani who'd come in from Brooklyn, "the date says 17 Tammuz."

"So?"

"So, that's a fast day. I think we'd remember if she died on a fast day." The seventeenth of Tammuz on the Hebrew calendar commemorates the breach of Jerusalem's walls before the destruction of the Second Temple and the Jews' exile to Babylon in 70 CE. Some people honor the day by abstaining from food and drink.

"She died on zayin, the *seventh* of Tammuz, not the *seventeenth*. The date is wrong!"

"Oh. Damn."

I pulled my father aside and alerted him to the problem.

"Eh, yes, Mamaleh, I can see that. I don't know how that could have happened."

"Aren't you the one who ordered the headstone? The one you asked me to write that epitaph for?"

"Oh. Well, don't worry, we'll fix it."

"Please Ta, she deserves to have the right date on her stone!"

The numbers seven and seventeen in Hebrew lettering are differentiated by only a tiny letter, yud, which looks like a "1." All that needed to be done was to leave the letter representing the

number seven and delete the extraneous yud. It was a simple fix
and one I hoped would happen quickly.

Before leaving the cemetery, everyone present searched for a
small rock to leave on the headstone, indications to future visitors that the person buried there was missed and loved. Every
time I've visited her grave since, the amount of rocks has grown.

Initially, I visited my mother's grave more often than I should
have, sometimes once a week. I ignored the Jewish custom to avoid
visiting the grave of a family member for the first year, choosing
my own comfort over the notion that my presence would make
it harder for my mother's soul to move on to the spiritual world.
A few visits after the unveiling, I saw that the yud had been filled
in with a putty close enough in color to the stone that unless you
were looking for it—which obviously I was—you'd never notice.
Finally, I thought, my father had put me out of my misery.

"I didn't do it, Geechee," my father confessed when I called to
thank him. "It was Dafna!" Why he sounded proud that his fiancée
paid to have his first wife's tombstone corrected was beyond me. If he
thought it would make me warm up to her more, he thought wrong.

My father and Dafna got married in early July. The third-time
bride wore a full-length white gown and a tiara encrusted with
jewels on top of a dark, shoulder-length bob—a wig she wore
in keeping with the tradition of some Jewish women who cover
their hair once married and continue to do so even after divorce.

Our rabbi suggested we arrive after the ceremony, assuring
us this was common practice for children of a bereaved parent
getting remarried. We waited at home playing a guessing game
of "what part of the chuppah do you think they're at now?"
until one of our mom's friends called to say the reception was
about to start. I piled everyone into the Caravan and drove the
few blocks to the Young Israel of Staten Island, the same shul
where our mom's funeral had been held. It wasn't in the same

sanctuary—her funeral was in an auxiliary space reserved for congregation overflow—but it was still the same congregation. I doubt my father and Dafna had considered this when booking the hall. He probably hadn't bothered to mention it to her. It was unintentionally, unnecessarily cruel. At four, Gita was too young to understand that her mother was being replaced. Miryam, Eli, Rivky, and I knew we had no say in the matter and although we resented her, we understood that Dafna was the best our father could do. He was an only child whose parents were long gone, and he needed someone by his side. And Dafna, who seemed to have come through her divorces with some financial stability, didn't need much more than that from my father.

The five of us huddled close together in our nice new outfits, all paid for by Dafna, and walked into an elaborate reception where my parents' friends did their best to pretend this wasn't deeply weird and painful.

Later that summer, I found a bunch of young women who, like me, observed Shabbat and kosher, and were looking for a fifth roommate to split the rent on an Upper West Side apartment, and moved in with them. The place had four bedrooms, two on the ground floor and a deathly spiral staircase leading down to two more on the basement level. The staircase was so narrow it was like spinning in place until you were finally downstairs, at which point you'd need a minute to regain your balance. My window looked at the concrete "courtyard" and got almost zero sunlight, but it was the biggest room in the place. With the slight raise I'd been given at my now full-time fashion job, I could afford to pay my rent and utilities myself. I was thrilled.

My dad loaded his borrowed station wagon with my garbage bags full of personal belongings and helped me move in. In the great tradition of first apartments, my furniture consisted of cast-offs from friends and family, including my mother's old oak night table, Suri's childhood desk, and a faux Persian rug my dad had held on to from his Manhattan showroom days.

During my first year on the Upper West Side, I attended close to a dozen of my friends' weddings and racked up quite the collection of bridesmaid dresses. By my sixth or eighth dress, a panic started to grow. Everyone seemed to be pairing off except for me. Even my younger brother, all of twenty-one, got married that year.

I walked up the aisle at his wedding, smiling deliberately with my head held high and looked straight ahead toward the chuppah. By community standards, I was a twenty-two-year-old motherless spinster at her younger brother's wedding, but I didn't want their pity and I didn't need their matchmaking services. I'd find a man, the right man, on my own. Eventually. I hoped.

Balancing my career ambitions with the mounting pressure I felt to get married while also keeping tabs on my sisters took up all of my headspace. The job I loved started to lose its luster. I couldn't see any more room for growth. My work environment became more and more stressful (think *The Devil Wears Prada*) until I reached my breaking point and walked out the door. I allowed myself one day of self-pity before calling a few friends for leads. Someone's friend's cousin worked for an ophthalmologist, and they were looking for front office staff and that's all you need to know about how we found employment in the nineties. It was a far cry from the glamorous world of making fabric swatch books and inspiration collage boards of my previous job, but the pay and benefits were great, and my boss was a religious Jew like me, which made it easy to take time off for Shabbat and holidays.

After ten uninspiring months of wearing a standard-issue white lab coat and helping senior citizens complete presurgical forms for their upcoming cataract procedures (did I mention how good the pay was?), I heard the fashion world beckoning me back. OK, so I beckoned the fashion world back with a phone call to my friend Edina. We'd worked at that first job together and she left shortly after me for the same reasons.

"Edina, get me out of here," I begged after describing the tedium of the medical office.

"Yo." (She was from Brooklyn and said "yo" with zero irony.) "I'm doing PR for a men's sportswear line now; you wouldn't like it here."

"OK, well if you think of anything . . ."

"Wait, I got it!" she said. I was excited before even hearing what it was she got. "Last week, I met an Italian dude who's setting up a showroom in midtown for a men's line called Energie. It's like Diesel, but no one's heard of it."

Menswear did not excite me. My heart belonged in womenswear. But there was more. "They also have a junior sportswear line called Miss Sixty and he mentioned they were looking for someone to run their PR and marketing. You'd be perfect. I'll call him and put in a good word."

A few days later, in a penthouse showroom with floor-to-ceiling windows overlooking Bryant Park, I sat opposite the man who would become the best boss I ever worked for. I'd be responsible for planning events in major US cities and wooing magazine editors to use Miss Sixty samples in their fashion shoots. Even better, *I'd* be wooed by ad salespeople from those same magazines, since I'd be deciding how to spend our advertising budget. I was hired on the spot. Like I said, it was the nineties.

I had my dream job, an Upper West Side address, and roommates who were all professionals climbing their respective corporate ladders. Best of all, they were all still single like me. This went a long way to counterbalance the pressure to get married, which had ratcheted up significantly since my brother's wedding.

My roommates were also a vital sounding board during the two-year period when I had back-to-back boyfriends, none of whom were even close to being *the one*.

In no particular order, there was Jack the day trader who liked to tell me how much money he earned, but insisted we always split the bill and, in the dead of winter, preferred walking thirty blocks to taking a taxi. Also, he spoke to his mom in St. Louis three times a day. Sometimes more.

Dov was a martial arts expert who was studying acupuncture and herbology. He was five years older than me and lived in his sister's converted attic in Brooklyn. We were friends who evolved into something more, who then evolved into nothing when I realized he wasn't going to resolve his love-hate relationship with Judaism any time soon.

Joey and I had a Hollywood-worthy meet-cute; he was leaving a physical therapy office while I was walking in for some neck pain relief. At my next appointment, I worked up the nerve to ask the receptionist about him and she handed me a scrap of paper with Joey's number on it—he'd asked her to pass it on to me. Swoon. He took me to dinner where we talked for hours and made plans for a second date the following week. I waited at home for more than an hour, but he never showed up. A few days later, I saw his name flash across my cell phone, but I didn't answer. I found a new physical therapist.

They couldn't have known it, but these men were all place-holders, practice boyfriends until the real thing came along. Perhaps I was their placeholder, too. It didn't matter. My mother once told me I'd know when I'd found *the one*, which meant I'd also know when someone wasn't the one.

When I visited my grandfather in Canarsie, I'd brace myself for his "Nu? So, vat's mit the dating?" I introduced him to several boyfriends, and he was always polite if not a little reticent. He only wanted to know which one I'd be marrying. After a breakup, he'd inevitably declare, "Good, that von vas a putz anyway."

"So, why didn't you say something, Zaidy? I'd have ended it sooner!"

"Vell, I'm not the von who has to marry him, you do."

He wanted to see me settled. It was almost like my mother's ghost was nudging him to nudge me.

One warm Friday night in September 1997, at a typical Upper West Side Shabbat dinner, I sat with a bunch of other singles crammed around a dining table that someone had inherited from their grandma, eating broccoli kugel, cranberry crisp, meatballs (no one was springing for a good cut of meat), and sweet and sour chicken. Most of us had grown up in homes that placed great emphasis on sitting down to Shabbat dinner with family. We'd heard our fathers make kiddush on wine and a different blessing on the freshly baked challah. Our parents laid their hands on their children's heads and blessed us. In the absence of that structure, Jewish young professionals sought each other out and created a new type of family with whom to celebrate Shabbat. These dinners, along with the Friday night prayer services at local shuls, doubled as our dating scene.

I looked around the table at the same faces I'd been seeing week in, week out at shul and parties, and felt utter despair. *Ugh, I'll just marry one of these idiots and be done with it.* I was all of twenty-three. By Orthodox Jewish standards, though, time was ticking. I was careening toward my expiration date faster than that nauseating free-fall ride at Six Flags. Another pressure point was my medical history. The breast specialist I'd been seeing annually had warned me of the risks of estrogen exposure given my family history of breast cancer. Pregnancy makes estrogen levels skyrocket, so if I was going to have kids, I was strongly advised to do so on the earlier side. High estrogen levels close to the age my mother was at diagnosis would be as risky as taking that Six Flags ride without wearing a safety harness.

The next day, my roommates Rebecca and Jen were hosting a small lunch in our apartment for an old childhood friend. The Upper West Side Shabbat lunch experience could range from eating deli sandwiches in your pajamas with your roommates to a buffet for twenty-five where every surface from the radiator to the bathroom sink was a potential place to perch your bowl of cholent. I'd had other plans, but bailed at the last minute, exhausted from having taken the red eye from San Francisco for a work trip. The table was set, the food my roommates had cooked Thursday night was warming on an electric hot plate, and I was growing impatient. And cranky.

"Do you guys mind if we get started? I just want to read and take a nap," I yawned, listing my two favorite Shabbat pastimes.

"Yeah, we're just waiting for Phil." Right. Phil. I had a vague recollection of Rebecca mentioning a guy she and Jen had grown up with in Lakewood, NJ.

"He was in Boston for college and just moved to New York for law school, so our moms asked us to invite him for a Shabbat meal," Jen explained, placing a floral arrangement on the new table runner she'd purchased. Jen was never off duty from her job at Ralph Lauren Home.

"More like *made us* invite him," Rebecca clarified. "He's like our kid brother."

While I was doing some mental math and arriving at the conclusion that this Phil was probably my brother's age, we noticed someone squinting and waving through the iron bars of our ground-floor apartment window. He had wire-rimmed glasses, perfect white teeth, and a buzz cut with wide mutton chop sideburns. *Strange* was the first word that came to mind. I'd never met anyone with such an extreme hair style; and I worked in the fashion industry. He definitely didn't look like the conventional Upper West Side guys I knew. Jen went to meet him at the door.

Phil apologized to Jen and Rebecca for being late, said he'd overslept and was tempted to stay in bed, but knew they'd report back to his mother and he'd never hear the end of it. "Oh, Jessica would have killed you for sure!" Rebecca agreed, laughing.

Turning to me he said, "Hi, I'm Phil by the way." Up close, his sideburns looked even more theatrical, but I also got a whiff of what I recognized to be Gaultier Le Male cologne. My favorite. *He could be one of your little brother's friends*, I reminded myself and replied, "Gila. Nice to meet you."

Over potato kugel and schnitzel, we swapped stories about the week; Rebecca, who worked in travel PR, vented about her controlling boss; Jen was happy that her late nights at Ralph Lauren had paid off and was getting recognition for the showroom display she created; and I offered some anecdotes about meetings with boutique owners on my recent visits to Miami and San Francisco.

Phil then turned to me and asked, "So, what do you do for fun?" His own recap of the week involved several late-night parties.

"Read," I yawned again, thinking there'd be no follow-up questions. I could practically hear my bed calling out to me.

"Who's your favorite author?" *A follow-up question that was neither "Where'd you go to college?" or "Where are you from?" How refreshing!* Phil now had my full attention; I noticed he was cute, mutton chops notwithstanding.

"Margaret Atwood, especially *The Handmaid's Tale* but I love all of her books." I was glad I'd changed out of the ratty sweatpants I'd slept in and into a flattering skirt/blouse ensemble I'd brought home from work. Something was beginning to simmer

between us when Rebecca, oblivious to our sudden, intense interest in each other, cut in.

"How was your birthday weekend?" she asked Phil while cutting up a pan of Duncan Hines brownies for dessert.

"Oh, it was *amazing*," he said, rolling his eyes. He'd spent
his twenty-second birthday weekend with his family and half
the congregants of their shul at an old run-down kosher hotel.
It must have been a Lakewood institution because he, Jen, and
Rebecca were cackling.

"Too bad we couldn't be there," Jen said unconvincingly, wiping tears of laughter from her eyes.

After lunch, Rebecca offered to walk with Phil toward his
dorm on W 60th Street. It would be a shame, she pointed out, to
waste a blue-skied autumn day.

"Anyone else care to join us?" she asked, digging around the
kitchen junk drawer for her sunglasses. Jen passed, choosing
sleep over sunshine. Our other two roommates followed suit. A
nap was now the furthest thing from my mind, and I tried to
sound nonchalant when I said, "Sure, why not?"

From the minute we headed out, Phil and I talked and laughed
nonstop while Rebecca trailed behind, lost in her thoughts and
still oblivious to the budding romance between her roommate
and a kid she grew up with. I, on the other hand, was keenly
aware of how quickly I was falling for this boy in motorcycle
boots and cargo pants. I'd never felt anything even close to this
with anyone else I'd dated. I was even starting to like those stupid
Elvis sideburns of his.

Shortly after walking past the Boat Basin on West 79th, Phil
realized he'd left his keys at our apartment. He asked if we could
all walk back and get them.

"Don't you have a roommate who can let you in?" I wondered.

"Yes, but I'd rather have my keys now, so I'll just walk you and Rebecca back home."

And that's when I knew: He felt it, too.

That night, a group of us went out and Phil joined. By 1:00 AM, our group had dissipated and gone off to their respective apartments, but Phil and I walked to the corner store where he bought me a Bacci chocolate and a diet Arizona green iced tea. He walked me home, but we had not yet run out of things to talk about. We sat out on the front stoop of my building, shoulder to shoulder.

"So. When was your birthday?" I asked, picking up on the conversation from lunch.

"It was just last week, September 14," he said, unwittingly setting my internal organs on fire.

That was my mother's birthday.

My mouth said, "Oh. Cool." But my brain was hyperventilating OH MY GOD THIS IS IT HE'S THE ONE YOUR MOM SENT HIM TO YOU YOU'RE TOTALLY GETTING MARRIED THIS IS JUST LIKE A MOVIE WOW YOUR PULSE IS MOVING PRETTY FAST YOU'D BETTER GET THAT UNDER CONTROL BREATHE BREATHE BREEEAAAATTTHHHHEEEEE.

"That was my mom's birthday," I finally managed in what I hoped was the voice of a normal person. "She died three years ago."

"Oh . . ." was all he said, but his eyes said more. *Oh. This is bashert. We are meant to be.*

Within weeks of our first encounter, we were already making plans for our future together. He brought me home to meet his parents, who were thrilled that their firstborn had met a woman as stubborn and driven as he was, but had hesitations about Phil getting married before he finished law school.

"I'm not waiting three years to get married," I told him over bowls of cereal at a New Jersey diner on our way back from Lakewood. "I earn enough to support us both."

"Gila," he said, reaching for my hands across the sticky Formica table, "if you're willing to give me a little time, I promise we'll build a beautiful life together."

His eyes were wide with hope, and I softened my stance for this boy who had my heart.

"OK. But not three years. Your parents will have to meet me in the middle," I smiled and tightened our interwoven grip.

My father loved Phil from their first handshake hello and, more importantly, so did my grandfather. The first time I brought Phil to meet my zaidy, we sat down to a heavy lunch of Babi Becky's notorious minestrone soup and despite my warnings that it would give him nuclear level gas for at least three days, Phil ate the bowl clean and asked for more while she watched him, beaming. He also brought *The New York Times*, bagels, and cream cheese from the city and a carton of Tropicana orange juice, not the generic brand they stocked in their 1970s yellow refrigerator. Two of Phil's grandparents were Eastern European Jews who'd also escaped the Nazis, so he understood how to speak to my grandfather about the old country and US politics, making sure to sprinkle in some classic Yiddish phrases. As we prepared to leave, my grandfather pulled me aside to give me fifty dollars and one of his signature brisk but firm hugs. He pulled back, looking me in the eyes as he nodded.

"So, Zaidy, what do you think of Phil?" I asked, already certain he approved.

"Mamaleh, vat can I say, you have more mazal than seichel!" he laughed. I shook my head, laughing, too. His comment that I had more good fortune than common sense referred to the string of questionable boyfriends I'd introduced him to before Phil came along, none of whom he'd liked. My grandfather understood better than most how important it was to have good luck and in his eyes, it was mazal that brought Phil to me. Having "more mazal than seichel" wasn't an insult—it was a blessing.

Eight months after first laying eyes on each other, we were engaged. Phil proposed to me exactly as I'd hoped he would: without any pomp or fanfare. In fact, it was while we were driving through the entrance of the Lincoln Tunnel. He reached into his pocket and pulled out a velvet box. "Gi, will you marry me?" he asked, eyes on a traffic cop whose sweeping hands directed us to merge left. I took the box from his outstretched hand, opened it, and removed the bezel set solitaire ring we'd chosen together, holding it up to the light before slipping it onto my finger. "I sure will, Philip Pfeffer!" I glowed, grabbing his face in both my hands and kissing him hard, nearly causing a collision.

A few weeks later, his parents threw us a huge engagement party in their backyard. While our guests clinked glasses and mingled beneath a white canopy tent, Phil's mom pulled me aside.

"So, daughter-in-law," she said, smiling, "we haven't talked about what you're going to call me." Until then, she was "Mrs. Pfeffer" to me. "You're welcome to call me 'Jessica,' of course, but if it's not too presumptuous, I'd love it if you'd call me 'Mom.'"

"Mom," I said, trying it on for size. "I like that! Mom it is." It had been years since I'd had reason to use the word, yet it felt natural coming out of my mouth. It felt good.

When I was little, I didn't dream of my wedding day so much as dreamed of my wedding dress. With a mother who'd studied at the Fashion Institute of Technology, it made sense that fashion design was second nature to me. My only use for Barbie dolls was as mannequins for my creations made from scraps of fabric I salvaged from my mother's sewing table. At thirteen, I started turning those scraps into hair scrunchies that I sold at school. At fourteen, I created a limited collection of denim skirts and t-shirts for a local Brooklyn boutique called Hooked on Juniors and for an entire week, my button and ribbon-festooned garments were on display in their bay window before selling out. This is why my wedding dreams never featured a groom or a chuppah or even a dance floor, just me in a white taffeta gown with a cinched waist, a hoop skirt the size of a circus tent, and puffy sleeves voluminous enough to stash a Volkswagen. It was the eighties! My notebook doodles were all variations of this dress. Sometimes the skirt would feature a lace overlay, sometimes embroidered seed pearls, but the theme was fundamentally the same: HERE COMES THE BRIDE.

My actual wedding gown bore no resemblance to the doodles of my youth. It was a spare, A-line silhouette of white organza over duchess satin with a waterfall of tiny silk flowers pouring down the back. My veil consisted of a single oversize piece of tulle draped from my head down to the floor. I looked like a ghost in love.

Aside from my mother's absence and Dafna's presence, our wedding was perfect. The chuppah was a tallis, which had belonged to Phil's belated grandfather, hung from the ceiling by invisible fishing wire. Pillars of twisted birch and white flowers stood at each of the chuppah's four corners.

Flanked by his parents who held white tapered candles to ward off the evil eye, Phil walked up the aisle, and took his place alongside his groomsmen. He wore a tuxedo under a white cotton kittel, a simple robe meant to symbolize purity and holiness. From behind an ivy-covered trellis, I watched my bridesmaids walk down in twos, followed by my siblings. First, Eli and his wife, then Miryam and Rivky in pale gray sweaters and silver ball gown skirts. Last was eight-year-old Gita, my flower girl, in a frothy white dress. I'd personally sourced all of their outfits. *Look at us*, I swelled with pride as they giggled down the white fabric runner, *as elegant and meticulously made up as anyone else with a mother.*

My dad insisted on Dafna escorting me with him. I was horrified. She didn't deserve the honor of ushering me to my wedding canopy. Plus, I wanted to minimize the number of photos she appeared in—with any luck, I'd be able to avoid putting any of her in our wedding album. In the end, my solution was to have her and my dad walk me halfway up the aisle. They then walked the rest of the way alone while I waited for Phil who came back down the aisle to pick me up. We entered our chuppah, a symbol of our future marital home, together.

Just before we took off, he leaned his head toward mine and whispered, "Here we go!" There we went, indeed, smiling like people who'd just won the lottery. Our guests, my mother's friends in particular, wept unabashedly.

The two years following our wedding were full of more joy than I'd experienced in my first twenty-five. We lived our best newlywed lives in a ground-floor apartment on West 93rd Street, directly across from the apartment I'd shared with my friends. A headhunter lured me to a new position at a kids' clothing company where I became the Director of Marketing and E-Commerce. I was ready for a job that required less travel than Miss Sixty, plus my new job came with a considerable salary bump and the chance to learn how to code just as online shopping was taking off. Phil graduated law school and passed the bar, both of which were reasons to celebrate, but I was excited for another reason.

"I'm so proud of you, hon, great job!" I squealed, hugging him tight. "And now… it's time to have a baby. Chop-chop!" Phil had been reluctant to start a family before he had a job. With the pressure of studying now behind him and an offer from a New York City firm, he was finally more than happy to comply. I was twenty-six and on a self-imposed deadline to be finished having kids by the time I was thirty-five, all to avoid that concerning estrogen spike given my family's medical history. I assumed thirty-five was enough years away from forty, the age my mother had been at her breast cancer diagnosis. Six weeks later, I was shrieking with joy and waving a positive pregnancy test in Phil's face.

We bought our first house, a three-bedroom ranch with yellow vinyl siding and an overgrown backyard in Highland Park, New Jersey, trading our dreams of city living for more square footage, a one-car garage, and as many Targets as I could drive to in our sensible family SUV.

In June 2001, after a thirty-six-hour labor, our son Ezra was born in the very same Upper East Side hospital where my mother had taken her last breath exactly seven years earlier. If she couldn't meet her grandson, I could take comfort in the knowledge that they'd occupied the same space, albeit in different millennia, and that her essence somehow lingered in the ether of that hospital and passed through him like a blessing for a good life.

4

days of onions

"You seem more relaxed," Phil noted as I unwrapped little Ezra's towel and blew loud raspberries on his freshly bathed belly. I loved the hysterical laughter this provoked from our fourteen-month-old son. It was the second day of our first family vacation.

"I *guess* so," was my reply, but said in an exaggerated singsong voice while maintaining eye contact with my giggling baby.

"Admit it, the trip was worth it. Look how much fun we're having."

I looked up at Phil and shrugged, reluctant to admit anything because I've always been stubborn. He knew who he married.

We were on the carpeted floor of a family-friendly hotel in Mont Tremblant, a Canadian town where Phil had tried to teach me to ski not long after we'd met. This was our first time there in summer and as we neared the end of our nine-hour drive from New Jersey, the air became thick with the scent of blue hyacinth, the view filled with endless poppies swaying in the breeze. I'd only ever seen Tremblant swathed in white and now I could make out hiking trails twisting around the green mountains.

It was Phil who thought a daylong drive with a fourteen-month-old would be a good idea. I'd have preferred to stay within an hour of our house—or better yet, not leave the house at all. Those same drives to Tremblant when we were dating, engaged, or newly married were filled with laughter, a highlight of our trips. But now? Motherhood had hit me like a Mack truck and my survival relied on predictability and routine. I was not the chill mom I'd always imagined I'd be.

Forty-eight hours earlier, Phil and I sat in the front seats of our car with Ezra strapped into his car seat in the back and the trunk was so crammed with stuff, we couldn't see out the back window.

Phil was buzzing, excited to take a much-needed break from his sixty-hour work weeks as a junior law associate.

I was a brick wall of tension.

We hadn't yet pulled away from the house when I started to list everything I wasn't sure I'd remembered to do. Turn off the oven? Stove? Iron? Did we have our passports? Did I remember Ezra's favorite stuffed doggie? Phil, who, unlike me, did not suffer from anxiety, gestured toward the dog in Ezra's lap.

Phil, bluffing: "Maybe we just won't go, then."

Me, calling his bluff: "Sounds good, I'll unpack!"

I was being ridiculous, and I knew it. I just needed a moment to get my head in the game. Growing up, we didn't take many family vacations, so I lacked some basic understanding of their importance to balanced living and good mental health.

I went inside to do a sweep of all the household appliances, hoping to justify my neurosis by finding all four stove burners on full blast. Unfortunately, all was in order. On our way up north,

Phil repeatedly asked me if I wanted him to turn around so I could check the house *one more time*.

Within an hour of our arrival, I'd set up Ezra's Pack 'n Play, highchair, and makeshift changing table. I then secured all electrical sockets and sharp furniture corners. The three of us set out to enjoy the fresh mountain air and postcard views from the cable cars. By the time we got Ezra to sleep that first night, I was relaxed enough to turn my attention to a pressing matter that Phil and I had been discussing lately: making a sibling for Ez.

If I wanted to be done having kids before I turned thirty-five, Phil and I were going to have to maintain a production rate of approximately one kid every two and a half years. Estrogen would give me children, but it could also kill me. Estrogen was my frenemy.

And now, two days into our trip, I was getting Ezra ready for bed when my cell phone rang. I flipped it open and was surprised to see my father's number on the gray, backlit screen. We spoke about once a week, usually on a Friday when I called to wish him a good Shabbos. It was a Tuesday.

"Hi, Ta," I answered, staring out the balcony window.

"Mamaleh," he rasped, sounding like he was fighting back tears.

Oh no.

"Gi," he tried again, "I have pancreatic cancer."

It was exactly ten years, almost to the month, since my mother had called me in Israel to confirm her diagnosis. Now I was in Canada receiving similarly grim news. Maybe I should stop traveling to foreign countries. Maybe I should stop answering my phone.

"Ta, what are you talking about?" He tried to steady his voice as he explained that a few days earlier, his skin had turned bright yellow. "Like a banana," Miryam later said when I called to press her for more information. "That's when I thought I should ask Bernie if he knew what was wrong." Bernie was an old friend who happened to be a doctor.

That got my attention. My dad wasn't a man who went to doctors. He didn't even have health insurance. "Too expensive," he'd say. "Besides, I'm perfectly healthy, I don't need it," completely missing the point of health insurance.

Bernie didn't charge him for the visit, which included a comprehensive blood workup. The results indicated that he likely had pancreatic cancer.

I knew only one thing about pancreatic cancer: The survival rate was low. By the time any symptoms presented, like, say, developing a complexion that would allow you to pass for a cousin of Homer Simpson, it was too late. This, combined with my family's survival track record, made for a grim prognosis.

"Oh my God, Ta, when can you start treatment?" I asked. Phil, pulling Ezra's pajama top over his head, was mouthing, "*What?*" I shook my head and listened as my father rambled on about his commitment to fighting his (fatal) disease.

"OK, Ta, we're heading home the day after tomorrow, and I'll come check on you. In the meantime, please get some health insurance," I begged uselessly. Who would insure a man who'd just been diagnosed with pancreatic cancer? I saw myself back in my Staten Island shul, crying at my father's funeral. I tried to push the thought away.

I hung up the phone and stood still, letting tears of frustration stream down my face.

Of course he had cancer.

That was what my family did; get cancer. They leave the front door wide open, saying "Right this way!" to preventable disease.

The anxiety that had melted away upon our arrival was now back with a vengeance. You wouldn't know it from my beaming face in our vacation snapshots, but I was consumed with dread for the rest of the trip. It didn't help that my mother's friend Elaine had called while I was packing, to ask if I'd add my father to my medical insurance.

"It's not my *insurance*," I said slowly, as if explaining to a toddler, "my plan is through my *company*. Because I am an employee of the *company*."

"But could you add his name to your insurance? Or could he use your insurance card for his treatment? You have the same last name, so . . ." She was desperate to help my father, but I wondered if she fully understood what she was asking me to do.

"Elaine," I said even more slowly this time, "that would be"— and I dragged this part out for emphasis—"*insurance fraud*."

A few days later, I found myself driving through Staten Island to see my dad. For the life of me I couldn't remember how I'd gotten there. My mind was adrift from the second I pulled out of our driveway and my body, on autopilot, navigated to the house where I was raised. My rolled-up windows were no match for the stench of the recently closed Fresh Kills landfill and I raced the last few blocks, mouth-breathing until I turned onto Rupert Ave. while Nelly warbled about how "hot" it was "in here" from my car radio. Even with the air conditioner on full blast, I was sweating, nervous to see my father.

When I arrived, the sight of him was alarming. He looked like a color-saturated, pop-art version of himself. His skin was undeniably yellow, as were the whites (yellows?) of his eyes. His irises, normally hazel, looked eerily blue against his skin. Only the milk glass coffee mug in his hand looked familiar. He was fifty-three, but his otherworldly complexion rendered him ageless, like an alien.

Reluctant to touch him, I gave my dad a quick, loose hug.

"I know, Mamaleh, I look terrible," he apologized. My throat tightened; I gritted my teeth in an effort not to cry.

"Oh, it's not so bad, Ta," I said, trying to comfort him. "It's kind of pretty, actually." He cocked his head to the side with an "aw, shucks" smile.

"Well, I'm going to see a specialist at Sloan Kettering this week, so maybe he can get me back to looking normal."

"You managed to get insurance then?" This was an encouraging new development.

"Elaine did, she's amazing. She contacted Bikur Cholim and they took care of everything," he said, shaking his head in wonder. Bikur Cholim, Hebrew for "visiting the sick" is also the name of a long-standing organization that provides unlimited support to people with medical problems. They managed to secure a top-tier plan with a major carrier.

"Incredible," I said, shaking my head. "Have you heard from Dafna since this started?" A few years into their marriage, disenchantment had descended upon the serial bride as she came to grips with my father's ever-worsening financial position and the reality that his children could not stand her. Attempts to coax Gita into calling her "Mommy" had failed. Her only child, a woman my age living in Brooklyn with two children, was in the throes of a bitter divorce, and Dafna had moved back under the guise of supporting her.

"She called yesterday to say she was sending a mover to get the rest of her things," he said, sighing before taking a long slow sip of his instant coffee. "I told her I might have cancer; she said she was sorry to hear it." He'd hoped to garner some sympathy, that she'd offer to help him through whatever came next. It didn't work.

"I'm sorry, Ta. You're really getting hit from all sides." I patted his shoulder.

"Eh, you know what I always say, Gi. 'Yom asal, yom basal,'"
he shrugged, using a favorite Arabic phrase. One day honey, one
day onions. "I guess I've had more than a few days of basal lately.
But that can only mean I'm due for a day of honey very soon."

The surgical oncologist recommended a major procedure called
a Whipple, which could increase the chance of his five-year survival to 25 percent by removing the head of the pancreas, the gall
bladder, duodenum, part of the stomach, and surrounding lymph
nodes. The remaining pancreas and digestive organs would then
be reconnected. The operation would take anywhere from four to
twelve hours. All of that for a mere 25 percent chance at survival,
but my father was undeterred. When it came to his prospects of
success in any aspect of life, he maintained a near delusional level
of optimism.

"Fuck this cancer. I'm gonna beat this sonafabitch, guys," he
announced, but his voice dropped really low when saying the
F-word. For a devoutly religious man who prayed three times a
day, made time for daily Talmud study, and followed a strictly
kosher diet, he cursed an awful lot. It was a quirk I found equal
parts endearing and confusing as a kid growing up with a mother
who often threatened to wash our mouths out with soap if we
so much as used the phrase "shut up." One time, I ignored her
dire warnings and said "doody" and found out she made good
on her threat. If you've ever wondered what a bar of Irish Spring
tastes like, please believe me when I tell you you're not missing
anything.

Two weeks later, Phil, my brother, and I hunkered down in a
waiting room at Memorial Sloan Kettering hospital with snacks,
books, and cell phones in hand to help pass the time. I'd just
discovered that operation "Make a Sibling for Ezra," which Phil
and I had launched in Canada, had been successful and I made

sure to have sleeves of saltines to quell the all-day nausea that had come surging back into my life. Hospital smells would only exacerbate my problem.

The surgeon promised to update us at the halfway point, so when he came striding toward us in his blue scrubs, we might have felt reassured to see him except that:

1. It had been less than an hour since my dad had gone into the OR and, accounting for the time it would have taken to prep and anesthetize him, it felt a tad early for an update.

2. The doctor's expression was less "update" and more "Houston, we have a problem."

He led with the good news: pancreatic cancer had been a misdiagnosis, so the Whipple procedure was no longer necessary. He then told us the bad news: my father had colon cancer. It had spread everywhere, including to his liver, which is why his skin had turned yellow.

"We had to stop the surgery and close him up. I'll refer him to a new oncologist, but as you probably know, colon cancer survival rates are much higher than pancreatic cancer, and given his young age, he should tolerate chemotherapy well enough. I'm sorry it's not better news."

He didn't look any happier to be delivering this news than we did to be receiving it. I had a violent urge to throw up and not just because of the gamey odor of rotisserie chicken wafting down the hall from the cafeteria.

Given how advanced his cancer was, my father was prescribed a high dose regimen of chemotherapy, which would be administered intravenously at the hospital on Manhattan's East Side. Miryam, by then twenty-two and working full-time in Midtown, often accompanied him to these sessions, which could last for hours. When she wasn't available, Phil or my dad's friends would step in. Unlike my mother, my father took his doctors' orders as gospel, never pushing back on any advice, often asking, "Is that the strongest medicine you have?" Perhaps *because* of my mother, he appreciated his mortality. And he wanted to live.

My dad tolerated the chemo fairly well. He'd always had a thick, dark head of hair, barely a gray to see despite his age and the many stresses he'd endured, and was as concerned about losing it as my mom had been. A silver lining was that colon cancer chemo is not the same as breast cancer chemo and their side effects differ greatly. My dad's hair color faded from black-brown to a translucent gray and thinned only a bit. His complexion had gone from yellow to plain old pale and the combined effect yielded a look I can best describe as "elderly apparition." He didn't want to go to shul each day wearing a baseball cap (I saw my father wear a baseball cap only once—when he was trying to make Gita laugh) or worse, have to affix his kippah to his bald head with tape. Because his hair remained somewhat intact, he managed to avoid both.

Sometimes on Sundays, Phil and I would take Ezra to visit him, and my father's face would light up, his voice becoming childlike at the sight of his grandson. With great effort, he'd lower himself to the living room floor to meet "Ezi" at his level and together they built towers and bridges out of colorful wooden blocks from a set he kept especially for this purpose.

During one visit, Phil asked my father how he was managing his taxi driving job while undergoing chemo. His CEO era was far behind him and these days, he ferried passengers in an old brown station wagon to and from airports in the tristate area.

"Oh, it's not too bad," he said with forced cheer. "We do what we've got to do, right, tatelah?" He directed the last part at little Ezra who was topping their tower off with a bright red cylindrical block. Watching them play made me think of an old photo of me and my dad riding a rocking horse together in that same room. I couldn't have been much older than Ezra when it was taken. My dad, still wearing his shirt and tie from a day at the office, would have been around my age.

Sometimes my dad and Gita would come for Shabbat and sleep in the finished basement of our three-bedroom ranch; my dad was afforded some privacy with the small bathroom Phil and I had installed downstairs, no small dignity given the bowel troubles his chemo caused. Late one Shabbat afternoon, I lumbered my way down the creaky wooden steps to the basement to see if they wanted something to eat, careful to hold the rickety handrail to steady my pregnant body.

"Hey guys, I've got bagels and tuna in the kitchen if you want," I said quickly, careful not to inhale. My dad's gas filled every corner of the basement, and I was grateful—for his sake and for mine, given my super ramped-up olfactory powers induced by pregnancy hormones—to be able to give him his own space. My father, a man who didn't own a pair of jeans or sweatpants because his quintessentially European ways dictated that he wear chinos at the very least and always a shirt with buttons, had to suffer this indignity while hoping to hold on to his life.

Gita was turning twelve in April of that year, so in January we started to think about how to celebrate her bat mitzvah and, more to the point, when. My father's treatment was failing; each scan showed tumor growth rather than reduction. On a cold Sunday morning in February, family and friends gathered for a party in the same shul basement, and catered by the same pizza store, as my bat mitzva a decade and a half earlier. Now though, I was attending with a twenty-month-old son while seven-months-pregnant with my second child.

Our decision to move Gita's bat mitzva date up had an unintended but crucial benefit. My grandfather, who had been in and out of the hospital with heart problems for years, was there. He must have held a torrent of mixed emotions in his heart at such gatherings, each one a reminder of the daughter he lost. As Gita danced and horsed around with her friends, I watched him taking in the festivities in his best polyester suit buttoned over a sweater for extra warmth. His eyes were watery, maybe from a cold draft slipping through a nearby window or maybe from taking in his daughter's collective legacy.

I hoisted Ezra onto one hip, no small feat given my protruding belly, and took him to join a dance circle with Phil and my father. My eyes kept drawing back to Gita, making sure she was having a good time. She knew too well why she was having a bat mitzva party at eleven years old. Miryam came rushing toward us, presumably to join the dancing, but as she got closer her face told me otherwise.

"I'm taking Zaidy to the hospital. Babi Becky found him in the bathroom saying he had horrible stomach pain. Don't tell Gita," she commanded, already heading for the door. A few hours later she called me from the hospital.

"It's his heart again and, this time, a hernia too," Miryam said, sounding resigned.

He passed away a few days later, this man who'd survived endless loss and grief and still held fast to his deep religious convictions. He never complained, lived modestly, and quietly supported his grandchildren's ambitions, stepping in whenever my father fell short financially. It was ironic that he had my father to thank for having been present at Gita's bat mitzva altogether.

My due date neared, and my monthly prenatal checkups became weekly visits, which meant I was taking a New Jersey Transit train to and from the city more often than I'd have liked. Although we'd moved to New Jersey before Ezra was born, I stuck with my OB-GYN practice in the city. Given the thirty-six-hour labor I'd had with Ezra, I didn't anticipate any problems getting to the hospital in time to have baby number two.

I started my maternity leave from the school uniform company where I'd been working for three years. My well-meaning boss was from a traditional family where women dropped out of the workforce after marriage. He was surprised that I'd returned to work after Ezra was born and was sure I would not after having a second child.

"You'll have two babies and a sick dad to juggle. And no mother to help you. I assume you'll want to stop working this time," he said, giving me an opening to bow out gracefully.

I took it as a challenge and assured him, like Arnold Schwarzenegger in *The Terminator*, that I'D BE BACK.

Two days before my due date, I drove myself to the city because I wasn't going to schlep my swollen body *and* my hospital bag on the train. I was done with the back-and-forth between New Jersey and New York and planned to demand that my doctor induce my labor. I was induced for Ezra's birth, because my amniotic fluid level was lower than my doctor would have liked and the induction made for a controlled, albeit long, birth experience. There was no sitcom-worthy scene of me waking Phil up at 2:00 AM, shouting, "Hon, I think it's time!" followed by a high-speed race to the hospital along the dark, empty streets. Phil, always the more adventurous of us, was hoping for a more spontaneous experience this time around. He left his midtown office to meet me for what I expected to be our final prenatal appointment for baby number two.

"I've got my bag in the car, and I want Dr. Larafin to send us straight to the hospital from here so maybe give your office a heads-up," I said before he had a chance to sit down.

"Oh, is that why you look so nice? Because we're seeing Dr. Larafin today?" he teased.

My doctor was a dead ringer for Noah Wiley from *ER* and, as if that wasn't hot enough, he was Jewish. Although I loved all three obstetricians in the practice, it's true that Dr. Larafin was the only one I went to the trouble of washing and blow-drying my hair for, *and* putting on a full face of makeup. I was also wearing my most flattering maternity dress, a light blue paisley wrap number that somehow, even at forty-weeks pregnant, made me feel like a supermodel. Never mind that my face looked like a balloon artist had gotten at it with a pump, or that my midsection was undulating as tiny, sharp elbows and feet poked around looking for a way out. Even Phil couldn't deny how gorgeous this man was and what a magnetic, calming manner he had.

"OK, everything looks good here, but you're not yet dilated at all, so go home and we'll see you in a few days," the doctor told us after examining me.

"Oh, I was, um, hoping you'd induce me, like with my first." I didn't want him to think I was pushy or anything. But I also wasn't leaving without getting what I came for. "I've got my hospital bag in the car, so, all good to go!" I continued, going in for the hard sell.

The two men exchanged a look. Phil shrugged as if to say, "I know, man, I'm married to her."

"There's no medical reason to induce you, but I can strip your membrane right now, which has a high chance of sending you into natural labor," he said, referring to a maneuver that involved him sweeping a finger between the thin membranes of my uterus and amniotic sac.

"OK, two questions: Will it hurt? And does it work?" I didn't mind pain, but I wanted to manage my expectations.

"It won't be pleasant, but it should work. Membrane stripping is my specialty," he said, smiling so his warm, brown eyes crinkled.

"Fine," I tutted. I was annoyed to have been denied my request to go immediately to the hospital and get a Pitocin drip. I'd already made arrangements for my babysitter to watch Ezra, had my bag packed and, most important, I looked good. I pictured myself looking like a new mom from one of those women's magazines, all dewy as my newborn and I gazed into each other's eyes.

I lay back down on the table, squeezed Phil's hand tightly, and felt a shock of pain strong enough to almost make me black out, during which I forgot to be cool and composed in front of Dr. McDreamy, and I howled like a wounded animal.

"You did great, Gila!" he said, removing his glove and shaking a slightly traumatized Phil's hand. "Call me at the first signs of labor and I'll meet you at the hospital."

Outside on sunny Lexington Ave., I unleashed the wrath meant for Dr. Larafin onto Phil. "Can you believe that guy? Ugh, I bet it won't even work and they'll end up having to induce me anyway. I'm going home," I said, already storming off to the parking lot.

"Maybe you should hang around in the city," Phil suggested. "We can go get lunch and walk around on uneven surfaces to get the party started."

"No, I'm going home to Ezi. You go back to work; I'll see you tonight."

"OK," he said in a way that told me it wasn't really OK, "I love you, but for the record, I think this is a bad idea."

A few hours later, while visiting my sister-in-law back in New Jersey, I started to feel a little crampy. Actually, more than a little crampy, as I blew hard, rapid breaths out of my mouth in an effort to lessen the pain. It wasn't helping.

I called Dr. Larafin, and by the time he came to the phone, I was full-on panting.

"I'll meet you at the hospital in a few minutes," he instructed, assuming I'd stayed in the city like an intelligent person.

"It may take me more than a few minutes to get there." I had doubted his magic hands and now he knew it. I was mortified. More pressing was the matter of getting to the hospital on the Upper East Side from central New Jersey—a drive that took at least forty-five minutes without traffic—during rush hour.

"I'll take you," she said, firing off instructions for her nanny before leaving her two young sons and loading me into her Toyota Camry. I was glad I'd left Ezra napping at home with a babysitter. "Call Phil and tell him we're on the way." We swung by my house where I grabbed my hospital duffel and told the babysitter I might be a while. As an afterthought, I grabbed an old bath towel to sit on in the backseat of the car, which turned out to be a wise move when my water broke like a dam halfway to the city.

On all fours with my head hanging out the window like a dog, I managed to brief Phil through my labored breathing, and he got to work, arranging police escorts to meet us on the turnpike. We lost some time when an ambulance pulled us over and a paramedic, yanking a rubber glove up to his armpit, instructed me to lie down in the back seat so he could deliver my baby and I was like "HELL NO." I had to sign a waiver of refusal of treatment before they let me go. Eventually, a New Jersey police car appeared and escorted us to the tunnel entrance where they told us the NYPD would meet us on the other side before sending us off. Every ounce of my energy was focused on breathing and keeping this kid tucked inside me. I'd read somewhere that if you're able to talk, you're not that close to push time so I blabbed incessantly, talking to my sister-in-law about everything I saw out the window. She was an adrenaline junkie, thrilled by her hair whipping in the wind as police sirens wailed around us. At the hospital entrance, an EMT transferred me onto a gurney and whisked me into an elevator while I screamed just like in the movies.

Dr. Larafin was standing there as the elevator doors opened and he glared at me, shaking his head as I was wheeled past him and moved onto a bed in a labor room. A few minutes later, a panicked Phil came running into the unit, grateful that I'd made it to the hospital safely, but furious that I'd ignored his advice to stay put.

"Get ready to push, Mom!" a nurse yelled and before my epidural had time to kick in, I pushed twice and out she came, all five pounds fourteen ounces of her. She was the first girl born in our family since my mom had died nine years earlier. We named her Faiga Leah, my mother's Hebrew name, and added on a third— Chaya, meaning "life"—as a protective mantle for our daughter.

Five months later, I went back to work, proud to prove my boss wrong but tired in ways I didn't know existed. I returned to the same schedule I kept after my first maternity leave: in the office three days a week. To keep myself awake during the twenty-minute drive each way, I relied on bladder-buster-size cups of iced coffee and smacking myself every few minutes. I considered quitting, but was terrified of giving up my career, of losing my identity to full-time motherhood. I was also terrified of getting into a car accident from chronic exhaustion. My boss could see I was struggling and had a suggestion.

"Would it be easier for you to work from home?" he asked. "I could have the IT department connect your home computer to our system." For a guy from such a traditional background, he was surprisingly feminist.

"That would make a huge difference, thank you!" I said, thinking that eliminating my commute was the answer to my problems.

This new arrangement lasted for six months before I came close to having a nervous breakdown. The produce aisle in Stop & Shop is as good a place as any to have an epiphany and it was there, next to a display of heirloom tomatoes, that I realized I had to quit my job. As I was pushing an overflowing shopping cart, I got a call from my coworker about a huge mess up in our warehouse that required my immediate attention. This was just the latest example of my home and work life blurring together and, as I abandoned my groceries to run home to my computer, I thought *No one is getting the best of me.* Phil often pulled all-nighters at work, and, unlike me, he was able to be fully present at his job. I wanted to be fully present for my job as a mother. We ran the numbers and agreed we could manage on his salary alone; I gave notice the next day and my relief was instant.

Becoming a mother of two while dealing with my own ailing father was a whirlwind unto itself. There was little I could do to comfort him outside having him to stay for Shabbat or bringing him home-cooked food, so I was proud to have given him two grandchildren. Sometimes I try to imagine what it must have been like for my mother to be a pregnant newlywed with a terminally ill mother. I wonder how she survived the sleepless nights of my first three months of life while helplessly watching my grandmother deteriorate. I think about whether the bliss of my arrival was enough to temper the pain of her death. Maybe naming me Gila, Hebrew for "happiness" or "joy," was meant to beckon some light into her darkness. Living up to my name, I brought my father joy through his grandchildren.

I called my dad a couple of times a week to check in, usually while I was with at least one of the kids. We both needed an infusion of joy into what were typically somber conversations. One day, nearly two years after he started his treatment, I dialed his number and tucked the cordless phone between my

ear and shoulder while feeding fourteen-month-old Lea some
yogurt. "What can I tell you, Gi," he said with a sharp exhale,
"the scans showed the goddamn tumors are growing. The good
news is they offered me a new chemo, something that was just
approved."

"That's so great, Ta," I said, putting the phone on speaker to
let him hear Lea's yogurty slurps and shrieks of delight.

"As long as they've got options to offer me, I'll take them. I
want to see little Ezi and Lea Pia grow up." What my father lacked
in good fortune, he made up for in high levels of endurance.

His stubborn nature combined with his tendency to view reality through a distorted lens served him well throughout his cancer
treatment. He had plenty of faith in his doctors but believed first
and foremost in the power of prayer. "Hashem is on my side,
Mamaleh." No matter how tough things got, my father felt that
God had his back.

I tried to yank back the blue plastic spoon clamped between
Lea's front teeth. It was her new favorite game. It made me laugh
and, in the high voice reserved for my babies, I cooed, "Zaidy has
Hashem on his side, did you hear, Lee Lee?" She laughed, loos-
ening her grip on the spoon, and I dug it back into the container.

"Also," he continued, "I read that sugar is fuel for cancer so
I'm eliminating all sugar from my diet. I'm gonna *starve* the sono-
fabitch out." He emphasized "starve" as if the mere mention of
the word could scare the cancer out of his body.

When I visited him a few days later, I found him sitting at the
kitchen table with a plate covered in powdered sugar. Next to
the plate was an Entenmann's box, the foil tray which had once
contained the preservative-laden cheese crumb cake (his favorite)
now empty.

"What happened to no sugar, Ta?" I asked, depositing Lea
onto his lap to free my hands to attack the sink full of dirty dishes.

"Oh, it's just once in a while. I need energy to do my job, you know. Driving a car service is more tiring than it looks!"

Miryam checked on my dad and Gita often, happier to visit now that Dafna was gone and no longer criticizing her every move. It was also a chance for her to catch up with Rivky, who commuted from home to Brooklyn College where she was a sophomore. Miryam would cook, do some light housework, and listen to Gita talk about school, her friends, and her upcoming eighth-grade graduation. She was also my primary source of *reliable* news about my father.

"He has a hernia, Gi and you're not going to believe this— wait, no, you'll have no problem believing this," she laughed into her cell phone while driving back to Brooklyn one night, "he saw a bulge sticking out of his abdomen and he's using a strap from a *camera bag* to hold it in!" She could hardly breathe from cackling so hard.

"Oh my God, Mir, please, did you tell him to go back to the doctor?"

"Of course I did, but you know Ta. He said, 'You don't need a prescription or a copay for a camera strap' and I didn't have the energy to argue with him."

Despite his MBA, deep down my father was still a farm boy from rural Hungary who valued fixing a problem with his own two hands, including, apparently, a hernia.

Not long after though, he was admitted into the hospital with a high fever and infection. Miryam was the only one with him when his doctors came to say that, after two years of treatment, they were out of options. I felt horrible I wasn't there to minimize the impact it had on my younger sister. Like me, Miryam was under no illusions that his cancer was curable, but she was closer to him than I was and much more forgiving of his shortcomings.

She cried when she heard the verdict and cried some more when relaying the news to me by phone from the hospital lobby. I started to well up, too, and offered to deliver the news to Rivky, Eli, and Gita. It was the least I could do.

"Poor Tati," she said, sounding exhausted. "You know what he said after the doctor left the room? He said, 'I had a good twenty-two years with Mommy, five wonderful kids. Maybe it will be OK on the other side,'" and the two of us bawled together.

Maybe there would be endless days of honey waiting for him there.

I dreaded having to explain to Gita what was about to happen, nostalgic for the time ten years earlier when my mother died and, at just three years old, she was blissfully unaware. Since Dafna took off, Gita and my dad had become an inseparable duo. When I told Rivky and Eli the sad but inevitable news, they took it as I would have expected. Like me, Eli, who was by then twenty-eight, had two young children, and we both counted our blessings that our dad had the chance to meet at least four grandchildren. None of us could believe that it was happening again, and that we were about to become orphans.

It was late November, just after Thanksgiving, which we didn't celebrate because it would have been too sad. My father demanded to be taken home for however much time he had left. "I don't want to go the way Mommy went, with the tubes, the machines, and the doctors," he said. He was in the hospital and getting weaker by the minute. "I just want to be in my own bed."

Phil took leave from work and my in-laws looked after Ezra and Lea for a few days. It was Phil who rode back to Staten Island in the back of the ambulance with my father, one of the last chances he had to show honor to his father-in-law of five years.

Phil later told me, "He kept trying to speak but his words were garbled. All the way home, he kept lifting his head to look out the window, pointing at signs and bridges. I think I heard him say 'Gowanus.'" That was the taxi driver in him talking. I have no doubt that if he could, he'd have grabbed the wheel from the ambulance driver and taken a better route, one that avoided tolls.

We hired a Hungarian hospice worker to care for him and preserve his dignity. She was focused, efficient, and stern with the rest of us, but softened when speaking to my dad in his native tongue. I am so grateful that this woman shielded me—all of us—from the frailties and decomposition I'd witnessed intimately with my mother. The sight of purple, bulging tumors down her back when she asked me to rub her skeletal neck and shoulders are burned into my brain and I wish I could delete those memories. My father flitted in and out of consciousness as friends and family stopped by to spend a few last moments with him. My mother-in-law brought freshly cooked chicken soup and sat by his bed trying to coax a spoonful into his mouth. The sight nearly cracked me in two and I hurried out of the room.

When he finally took his last breath, about an hour after Shabbat ended, Rivky, Miryam, Eli, Phil, and I were surrounding his bed. We opened the window a crack to allow his spirit an exit path as we listened to his shallow breath go from a rattle to nothing. Gita, however, was not there. We collectively encouraged her to go on her freshman Shabbaton, a school weekend away, as any normal thirteen-year-old would. It had been tough enough to start high school with no mother and a sick father. Gita often avoided discussing her home circumstances altogether. We never intended for her to miss the moment when he finally did go, although it was a mercy. The rest of us were adults; even Rivky was already twenty. Gita was barely a teenager.

Miryam's friends arranged to have Gita brought home early and, when she found out our father was gone, she was furious, her fiery red mess of hair slicing behind her as she bolted to her bedroom and locked herself inside. Later, we learned that she went there to retrieve a small suitcase from under her bed. The case was filled with tapes she'd made of conversations with my dad over the past year and some sweaters of his she'd squirreled away. She sat playing them one by one on a hand-size recording device, bathing herself in the sound of his voice and the musty scent of Irish Spring soap on his sweaters. She'd been anticipating his death as much as I had and that was sadder than losing my dad in the first place.

My father's funeral took place at a little shul up the street from our house where my family prayed when I was young. Its congregation was composed largely of Hungarian immigrants like him. Although my siblings and I eventually moved to a more modern local shul, my father remained loyal to a house of worship where the rabbi spoke only in Yiddish; it reminded him of his roots. The only immediate family, therefore the only mourners, at my father's funeral were me and my siblings. The five of us sat shoulder to shoulder in the front row of the men's section, Gita in the middle wrapped from either side in Miryam and Rivky's arms. At my insistence, a special accommodation had been made for the four sisters to sit in the section typically reserved for men. As the oldest living member of the family, I was calling the shots and if the rabbi wanted to honor my father in his sanctuary, he'd have to meet my terms. The women's section was upstairs, and I refused to be a remote spectator at my dad's funeral. I'd also gotten word that Dafna would be sitting up there. At various points throughout the service, we saw her pinched face peeking down from behind the lace curtains.

Miryam and I wrote a speech that Eli delivered. I'd have done it myself but sitting in the men's section was as far as I could push my luck. Unlike the rabbi officiating at my mother's funeral, this one did not grant me permission to speak before a room full of men.

Here is our tribute to our father: He was full of childlike wonder and optimism when his odds were poor. He loved cold beer but hated cold weather. He was charitable to the bitter end, giving even when he himself was in need. He celebrated his children's successes like they were his own and lived for our mother during their short years together. The love of his life was the land of Israel and it had been his unfulfilled dream to live there.

We tore our shirt collars for kriya and walked through a parted sea of our crying friends, out into the unseasonably warm December sunshine. My father's coffin was placed into a waiting hearse, and we followed it back down the block to our house. The five of us ate our symbolic hard-boiled eggs at the kitchen table before Miryam, Rivky, Gita, and I took our places on the low chairs opposite guests already waiting to comfort us, while Eli and Phil went back outside to a waiting car. They were honoring my father's final wish by flying to Israel to lay him to rest in the cemetery where his father was buried. Less than thirty-six hours later, they'd be back in New York and Eli would take his place beside his mourning sisters.

This shiva felt different to the one for my mother. It was smaller, more intimate. With the exception of Gita, who preferred to receive her throngs of friends in the privacy of her bedroom, we all sat together in the living room. We had no choice, really. Now we were the adults and all of the condolence calls, whether by our friends or those of our parents, were for us. I felt most comforted on the days that Phil brought Ezra, three, and Lea, twenty months, to the shiva house and Eli's wife brought their two sons. The four cousins tore through the kitchen, dining room, and living room on a loop, reminding me of the Friday nights I'd spent doing the same with Eli and Miryam when we were little. I remember Gita doing the same at my mother's shiva and my heart hurt when I realized she had been the same age as my Ezra.

Our third night of mourning coincided with the first of Chanukah. My siblings and I were self-conscious as we excused ourselves to the dining room to light my father's silver menorah. We mumbled the blessings on lighting Chanukah candles but skipped the traditional songs and struggled to contain our nervous giggles at how absurd it all felt. The living room was full of people pretending not to watch us. Depending on your perspective, we must have made either a pitiful or awe-inspiring sight. My friends brought beautifully wrapped Chanukah gifts for my kids, knowing I wouldn't have thought to go shopping during my father's final days. It was one of a thousand meaningful ways in which they showed up for me.

If my mother's death was followed by any administrative tasks, I was largely oblivious because my father handled them. This time there were mountains of paperwork, both relating to the "estate" (lol) and Gita who was a still a minor. My father named me and Eli as her co-guardians, roles we willingly took on. There were legal fees, court appearances, and something called "guardian ad litem," a person whose job it was to make sure that Eli and I were not taking financial advantage of our sister. His fee was ten thousand dollars for doing absolutely nothing so if anyone was milking my sister for money, it was that guy. Privately, we referred to him as the "guardian ad nauseam." There was the sale of our childhood home and the bleak realization that it had been leveraged to within an inch of its life. Although my father was fond of pointing out that the house was worth ten times what he and my mother had bought it for in 1975, insisting that when the time came for us to sell, it would provide nicely for us, he neglected to mention the unpaid mortgages and threats of foreclosure.

Credit card companies chased us via our estate attorney, hoping we'd settle our father's debts. "I received another letter from a Visa card your dad opened last year. He owes close to two thousand dollars on this one. Would you and your siblings care to settle that?" Calls like this one from the attorney became the norm.

"Are we legally obligated to?" I'd always ask.

"No," she'd say, "but some families choose to settle the debts of the deceased."

"Can they come after our personal assets?"

"No, these debts don't transfer to next of kin."

"Then absolutely no is my answer." It was "no" every time she called with a new collection letter.

Even more galling was the stream of credit card *offers* that continued to arrive in our mailbox long after he was gone. Credit card offers for a dead man who had horrible credit. The American Dream, indeed.

At thirty, I was now the matriarch of my family and found myself feeling more protective of my sisters. Gita moved into Eli's house (fewer rules, more fun, she reasoned) and Rivky moved in with me and Phil. In rebuilding our family through the next generation, I began to pay even closer attention to ways in which we could reverse the cycle of early death that had been trending so far. As the oldest, it would be up to me to carve a path toward prevention.

Sometime between Phil taking his leave from work and my father coming home from the hospital for the last time, I got pregnant with our third child. In fact, I was pregnant during shiva but didn't know it yet. My father's illness, I realized, began with one pregnancy and ended with another. If that isn't the circle of life embodied, I don't know what is.

When I think of my father, my mind goes straight to a weekday in early September a few months before he died. While Lea napped and Ezra was in preschool, my dad drove out to visit me. It was his last visit to my house. We sat opposite each other at my small kitchen table, steam from our hot drinks (coffee for me, instant Tetley tea with lemon juice for him) curling up into our faces. He blew on his mug for a few seconds before mumbling the bracha of shehakol under his breath, a blessing designated for beverages and foods that don't grow from the ground. He'd recently taken to reciting these blessings more slowly and clearly, with great emphasis on the final few words. Holding his kippah to his head with one hand, he chanted them with the awareness of a man who knew that his opportunities to make brachot and to enjoy the simple, human pleasure of consuming sustenance of any kind would soon be gone, even if the brave face he wore for the rest of the world suggested otherwise.

". . . shehakol nehiyah bedivaro!" he finished.

I answered with "Amen" and he raised his mug to me.

"L'chaim, Mamaleh" he said, and he meant it. To life, indeed.

"L'chaim, Ta." I wondered how much more *chaim* he had left in him. He was still receiving chemo, which gave him a lot of hope he could beat his cancer.

"Will Phil be home for Shabbos?" he asked me. Phil was working on a seemingly never-ending trial in Washington, DC, where he stayed all week. Mostly he made it home in time for Shabbat, but now, as the sun set earlier and the days grew shorter, it became more difficult for him to leave DC early enough to make it home in time.

"I think so, that's the plan anyway," I answered.

"It can't be easy for you, Geechee." He hadn't used this term of endearment in years. Until that moment, I hadn't realized I'd been missing it. "I know it wasn't easy for Mommy when you kids were little while I was on the road so much. She was really something, your mother. She was tough."

On a perpetual quest to attain financial security and grow each new business he started, my dad would take trips to a major department store in Columbus, Ohio, and parts of the south, always toting a case full of his home goods—tablecloths and matching cloth napkins, placemats, and napkin rings—and accumulating as many orders as he could. There were never enough orders and ever-slimming margins of profit, and he struggled to retain customers, slashing his prices to nearly below-cost. I have many childhood memories of him calling from a motel room somewhere, speaking briefly with each of us kids before asking to speak to my mom. He'd debrief her on the day's haul while we watched her face for signs of hope that he'd gotten a significant order. All I ever remember seeing was a worried scowl.

"Yeah . . . I guess I never really thought about how much Mommy did for us on her own while you were away. Believe me, I understand now!" I felt myself choke up at the memory of her, at the intensity of discussing her with my dying father. I took a big gulp of coffee, swallowing my tears as well.

"The truth is, Ta, I'm OK with how things are. Phil busts his ass at work—you know he wants to make partner, and this is what he has to do to stay in the running—and I bust my ass at home, and I love being a mom. I think I'm good at it. One day I'll get back to my career, but for now my energy and attention go to my kids. I'm lucky I get to do that."

Tilting his head to one side, he looked at me with squinted, appraising eyes.

"You know what, Geechee?" he asked, after a few silent moments, "You are a real pragmatic bitch."

I think he meant it as a compliment. I certainly took it as one.

5

outsmarting my genetic destiny

Eleven years after my mother died, when I was thirty-one, I learned that a simple blood test could confirm whether I was a carrier of a BRCA gene mutation. Named for the first two letters of "breast" and "cancer," a positive result would place my odds of developing breast cancer at 87 percent. As an added bonus, BRCA carriers have a 66 percent chance of being hit with ovarian cancer. Those sound pretty high until you consider my insanely strong family history of cancer, which cranked my risk up even further. A blood test would be nothing more than a formality, a scientific breakthrough to tell me what I instinctively knew. I would 100 percent be BRCA positive.

It was 2005 and genetic testing was far from commonplace. The famous Human Genome Project, an international effort to generate the first complete sequence of the human genome, had only recently achieved its goal by producing a sequence that decoded 92 percent of human DNA. There was growing buzz around mainstream genetic testing and although we were still years away from at-home spit tests like 23andMe or Ancestry.com, this development could tell me exactly what my body was up against. After a decade of playing defense, I'd finally have the chance to shift to offense. I could see a path to reversing my family's health trajectory.

Pregnant with my third child and sick of everyone in my family dying too young, my self-preservationist instincts went into overdrive. I already thought about my own mortality way more than your average thirty-year-old, but my obsession didn't stop there. I had my younger sisters and baby daughter to worry about, too. Because my sisters were still children when our mother died, the primary impact on them was that it rendered them motherless. For me, an adult, it was a wakeup call to get ahead of breast cancer. As the family matriarch, I felt a responsibility to take preventative measures not only for my own sake, but to set a good example for my siblings.

Shortly after I learned about genetic testing, my friend Stephanie told me she was scheduled to have a procedure called a prophylactic double mastectomy. That's a lot of syllables which amount to electively removing healthy breast tissue before cancer can take root. It was the first I'd ever heard of it and my immediate reaction was *I want that*. Reconstruction is usually done at the same time, unless a woman chooses to "go flat." Unlike the modified radical mastectomy my mother eventually underwent, the prophylactic version leaves the outer skin and sometimes the nipple and areola intact. It would be years before Angelina Jolie would make "prophylactic double mastectomy" a household phrase by writing an opinion piece in *The New York Times* about her choice to have the same procedure.

Stephanie and I met when I moved to Highland Park a few years earlier. Our kids were around the same ages, and we were both stay-at-home moms and active volunteers at school. We also had a family history of breast cancer in common, but her mother, who'd been diagnosed in her twenties, had caught it early and survived. By the time Stephanie told me about her upcoming mastectomy, she had already tested positive for the BRCA1 gene.

I went to visit Stephanie while she was recovering at home. My intention was to fulfill the mitzvah (good deed) of Bikur Cholim (visiting the sick), but it was also a reconnaissance mission. Other than a dental implant, I'd never had surgery and came armed with a million questions. How long was the operation? Had she had any reaction to the anesthesia? How much pain she was in and where? Did her new boobs look natural? And most important of all, on a scale of one to infinity, how relieved did she feel now that breast cancer was no longer a threat?

I knocked on the door and went inside as I announced myself.

"Helloooooooooo! You have a visitor!" I sang as I walked across the foyer. Her mother greeted me and pointed to the living room. "How's she doing?" I mouthed while unzipping my coat. She gave me a double thumbs-up, touched her palms together and looked heavenward. "Thank God," she said quietly.

"So?" I asked Stephanie as I plopped my pregnant self down on the couch, careful not to disrupt the intricate network of tubing that stuck out of her from all angles. All of my questions rolled into one: *So??*

"I'm OK! The pain meds are working, and my back is pretty sore, but mostly I feel relieved. I'm telling you, Gi, it's like a weight's been lifted. No more worrying. I'm free!" She beamed, all dimples and shining eyes.

She showed me her post-surgical sites, like a guide preparing a tourist for a hike through rocky terrain. Her chest was wrapped many times over in white gauze and clear plastic bulbs the size of lemons hung off tubes on either side of her rib cage. They were filled about a third of the way with a viscous, rust-colored liquid.

"Surgical drains," she explained, giving each one a little flick with her fingers. "They collect the extra blood and other fluids to stop them from accumulating in my body. I have to dump the contents a couple times a day and keep track of how much comes out to make sure it's less each time." She showed me a little notebook with a list of dates and measurements in decreasing amounts. "It's a little gross, but they're only there for a few more days, until they stop filling up with gunk."

"More like a *lot* gross," I said, recoiling slightly, which got a laugh out of Stephanie. I'd been peed on by my kids and caught their vomit in my bare hands without batting an eye, but medical gore made my insides churn.

Of the several options for reconstruction, she'd chosen silicone implants with an overlay of muscle taken from her upper back to give her "foobs"—fake boobs—a more natural look. "All I have to do is sit on my couch propped up with these pillows, some physical therapy to regain range of motion in my arms, and I'll be good as new," she reassured me. "Better, even."

During my next prenatal checkup, I asked my doctor to arrange a BRCA test. The OB-GYN practice had started to see an uptick in requests for this type of blood test. She agreed that for me it was a no-brainer.

"I'll make sure to have the test kit here for your next check-up," she said. "But are you sure you want to do this while you're pregnant?" She was concerned about the psychological toll of potentially finding out I was a carrier at a time when I was already hormonal enough. My doctor was cautious but never alarmist. It was hard to say how old she was. Her wiry gray hair was always pulled back into a messy ponytail, and she favored socks with Birkenstocks and rimless glasses which probably added years to her actual age. What mattered to me was that she'd been in the expectant-mother game for a long time.

"Absolutely," I said without reservation. Whatever the test results, I was already plotting my next preventative steps.

"Have you decided what to do if it turns out you're BRCA positive?" she asked, wheeling her little stool over to her desk to make some notes in my chart.

"Either way, I'm getting rid of these," I announced, grabbing a swollen breast in each hand. "No question. I don't want this threat looming over me anymore."

"OK then, I'll see you next month and we'll get you tested."

Rather than go through my insurance, I paid four hundred dollars to test with a private lab. The cost seemed astronomical but worthwhile given that it was still unclear whether my health insurance company would regard a genetic mutation as a pre-existing condition and deny me coverage. In my eighth month of pregnancy, my ob-gyn delivered the results: I was BRCA1 positive. She was devastated on my behalf. I was not. I felt validated, puffed up with the smug satisfaction that comes with being right. Now I could turn my attention to planning my double mastectomy.

Shortly after receiving my unofficial welcome into the "very high-risk club," I learned that the BRCA1 gene was discovered in 1994, the year my mother died. She was as much a victim of bad timing as she was of bad genetics.

My ob-gyn referred me to Dr. Giannaros, a breast cancer surgeon at a top NYC hospital, for close monitoring and to plan my eventual preventative mastectomy. She was accustomed to seeing patients in their fifties and sixties but had recently started to see younger women like me who were on a search-and-destroy mission against hereditary cancer. I wouldn't be the only thirty-one-year-old to seek out her expertise, but I was still far from the norm. During our first meeting, Dr. Giannaros went over my various options, from the minimally invasive to the extreme.

"Self-exams, of course, are key and coming here twice a year for me to do a manual exam is important, too," she began. "Annual mammograms and ultrasounds are a must, and some women opt to take a medication called tamoxifen as a precaution." Dr. Giannaros explained that tamoxifen was an estrogen blocker that is effective in reducing cancer risk. These were all commonly used methods of prevention for high-risk people, but for me, they were not enough.

"A double mastectomy would provide you with the most protection, but the other options are good, too. I don't want you to feel you have to take the most drastic route," she said. But I was already shaking my head, palm held up.

"I'm not taking any chances; I'm going all the way."

I was determined to have the surgery, but it would have to wait until I was done having kids—and, at eight-months pregnant with my third, I wasn't done just yet.

In August, I pushed out a seven-pound-eight-ounce baby boy. We named him Natan after my grandfather who had passed away while I was pregnant with Lea. My grandfather, Natan "Norman" Lerner, knew firsthand how critical good fortune was to survival. He never spoke of the horrors he endured at the hands of the Nazis, but I knew from my mother that he'd escaped during a death march at nineteen years old. The SS guards wore deep hoods to shield themselves from the driving rain, but they also obscured their peripheral vision. My grandfather took a chance and ran. He didn't stop until he reached a barn where he lived in secret among farm animals until an American soldier found and liberated him weeks later. Our Natan—Tani, as he was known from the start—was here because of my grandfather's audacity. We all were.

All four of my grandparents eventually made it to Brooklyn and started from scratch. They grew families, sent their children to Jewish schools, and held fast to their faith. It was the ultimate revenge against an enemy who sought to obliterate them. They taught us that life moves forward even after the worst has happened. There is nothing more Jewish than defying a traumatic past by rebuilding and thriving.

There's also nothing more Jewish than transitioning from a Holocaust story into one about a wedding.

In late December, Rivky, twenty-one and a recent college graduate, got married to a quiet, scholarly boy of twenty-two. He was one of seven children and, like her, seriously committed to Judaism. She was the first of us to get married since we had become orphans and as a result, I felt more maternal to her than sisterly. The wedding took place on the second night of Chanukah.

"One Chanukah we're sitting shiva and the next we're at Rivky's wedding," I noted to Miryam. We stood in our satin gowns, emotions running high as we watched our younger sister, resplendent in white lace, pose for the photographer. Miryam and I dabbed our eyes with tissues, trying to keep our mascara intact.

"I know, right?" She sniffled. "Like Tati would say, 'Yom asal, yom basal.'"

Eli and I walked Rivky up the aisle to the chuppah where her groom stood waiting for her. Our parents' friends wept silently but I felt joyful, defiant of our painful past as I ushered my sister into a better future.

Every time I thought about scheduling a date for the surgery, I'd find an excuse to delay. I was finding it much easier to be brave with my words than with my actions. I reasoned that at thirty-two, I was still eight years away from the age my mom was at diagnosis. I still had time.

"I feel like something's missing," I said to Phil one Sunday while throwing away Tani's last empty can of Similac. He was a year old and had moved on to whole milk.

"Something like . . . ?" he prompted me, unclear on where I was going.

"More like some*one*. A fourth kid. I can't explain it, but that's what's missing." I didn't add that this would also buy me another year and a half, minimum, until I had to really think about having that mastectomy.

When we were newlyweds, Phil used to say, half-jokingly, that he wanted ten kids. "Our own baseball team," was how he put it. Not being sporty myself, this prospect didn't appeal to me. Now, three kids, a mortgage, and an intensely demanding career later, he realized that when I repeatedly said "That's never going to happen," I was being sensible. But four, a nice even number, sounded good to him, too.

Dr. Giannaros recommended I have an MRI before trying to conceive. For more than a decade, my prevention protocol had consisted of self-exams, semiannual checkups and, from the age of thirty, mammograms and breast ultrasounds. The key to early detection was using a variety of detection methods and now we were going to throw an MRI into the mix. Each diagnostic method viewed my breast tissue from a unique angle and all combined to form a crack team of investigators leaving no stone (duct?) unturned. If there was a way to turn my body inside out to get a closer look, I'd have done that, too. The results of my MRI came back clean and within a few weeks, I was pregnant again.

Akiva, aka "Kivi," was born in June 2007, thirteen years almost to the day of my mother's death. I was still measuring time using that metric. It was impossible not to.

Kivi was the quintessential youngest child, fawned over and indulged by all of us. With my three older kids, I sometimes begrudged bed and bath-time rituals, but that became my favorite part of the day with him. Rather than place Kivi in his crib at bedtime, I'd sit in a rocking chair with his warm body against mine and hum into his curly head on my shoulder until I heard his gentle snoring. I willed time to slow down so I could savor each second of his babyhood.

While I was pregnant with Kivi, Miryam—who, like me ten years before, was at the mercy of matchmakers who didn't see her for the treasure she was—met an adorable guy named Mikey, who was a perfect fit for her. It was love at first sight for my whole family. We'd never encountered anyone quite so mild-tempered, and he was sporty, too, an adjective that described absolutely no one who shared our DNA. We were thrilled when they got engaged, excited to be linked to his clan of loving parents and three older siblings, all of whom were already married with kids. For the second time in my life, at thirty-three, I'd be stepping in as the mother-of-the-bride and this time, I'd be doing it with a two-month-old baby in tow.

Once again, Eli and I escorted our sister up the aisle to her chuppah. By then, our dad had been gone nearly three years.

I don't know many mothers-of-the-bride who sit hooked up to a breast pump while having their makeup applied or can feel their boobs fill with milk on the dance floor. It could have been the postpartum hormones, or my shapewear cutting off my circulation, but my emotions jerked me between tears and laughter the whole day. Throughout the night, my role kept shifting from sister to mother of little kids, to mother of my sister. It felt like a privilege, but it was overwhelming.

When we celebrated Kivi's first birthday, I still hadn't scheduled my surgery. I was playing a math game . . . if my mom was diagnosed at forty and I was only thirty-three, I still had tons of time. I should mention that I'm terrible at math.

It wasn't the prospect of a long, painful recovery that made me procrastinate, nor the inevitable scarring. It was my molten hot anxiety born of an overexposure to loss and poor outcomes. There's a word for what I was: a catastrophizer. I was afraid of something going wrong, of dying on the OR table, a translucent version of myself floating above my corpse saying, "Only *you* could die trying to save your own life. Loser." Plus, there was the fact of having four very small kids, being a stay-at-home mom, and an inherent belief that no one could possibly replace me while I recovered. A catastrophizing control freak. That was me.

It was our decision to move to London for Phil's job that finally pushed me to schedule a date. Over the course of our marriage, Phil occasionally proposed a possible move to the UK to better serve a large, London-based client. Phil's mentor had moved his family there for a few years as had others on his team. Knowing it would be a good career move to follow suit, he hoped I'd agree to go, too. Here's how those conversations went:

"Hon, it would really be a good idea for us to consider moving to London, just for a few years," he would say, knowing full well that his wife couldn't take her small children to the park without a diaper bag full of backup clothing and enough food to last for three days in the event they found themselves trapped in the shelter at the top of a slide. My brain could not compute what a move to another country would entail with—depending on when Phil was asking—one, two, three, or four kids.

"I'm not going anywhere, you do what you've gotta do," was my constant refrain.

"OK," he'd soldier on, "not now, but, like, someday in the future? It would be such a great experience for the kids, too. Just think about it." I did not think about it. Remember, I didn't want to take a family vacation to Canada with one child, why in the hell would I agree to move overseas with several of them?

But Phil was persistent. Eventually, I realized that if we were going to do this, it would be best to move while the kids were young, which finally led me to say, "OK, hon, let's go to London." Somehow, an adventure and a change from our small, suburban corner of the world sounded right, even if it wracked me with guilt about leaving Miryam and Rivky. One upside was that living in London would mean we were closer to Gita, who'd decided to pursue her degree at a Tel Aviv–based university. Our choice would disappoint Eli, too, but I didn't feel protective of him the way I did my sisters. We'd have more than a year to plan and find schools for the kids, and I deluded myself into thinking that would be enough time for my siblings to get used to the idea of us leaving.

Phil and I decided we'd go in August 2009, just before the new school year. I wanted to give myself enough time to fully recover and show up in London as the most confident version of myself, so I'd have to book my surgery well before then. I wanted the freedom to choose how and when to share my story with the people in my new life. Maybe I would, maybe I wouldn't. But with no outward signs of what I'd been through, the narrative would be mine to control.

A date for surgery was finally set: November 19, 2008. Per hospital policy, I was required to undergo a psych evaluation with a hospital social worker to ensure that I was of sound enough mind to decide to have elective surgery. There are lots of good reasons to opt for "medically unnecessary" procedures, self-esteem and confidence being among them. At thirty-four, my view on plastic surgery of any kind had always been a hard pass.

Having said that, once I was already going under general anesthesia for a lifesaving procedure, I thought I might as well have the cosmetic part, too. I'd grown four humans in my body in under six years (way to go, body!), and with each birth I retained a bit more weight, a greater distance from hip to hip, more sagging abdominal skin that looked like a deflated balloon. Why not tighten up my breasts and stomach for the price of an insurance copay?

My breast reconstruction options were as follows.

- Silicone implants, which I rejected outright for two reasons: I didn't want foreign objects in my body if I could avoid it and also, the implants are done in stages with tissue expanders over the course of months and no thank you to additional procedures. I wanted to get this over with and never have to think about it again.

- Hybrid of implants plus back muscle as an overlay which seemed like the worst of both worlds. On top of having implants, I'd have chunks taken out of my back and I couldn't wrap my head around having to recover from surgery on my front and back at the same time.

- A TRAM flap*: stomach fat and muscle are tunneled up through the midsection and into the chest where they are

---

* Today, TRAM Flaps are rarely used; they've been replaced with the less invasive DIEP Flap, which had just become available when I was researching my options. For me, it was too new and the procedure took much longer than the TRAM, which would leave me under anesthesia for more time than I was willing.

shaped into boobs. It's a more invasive surgery with a longer recovery time, but it would also mean the reconstruction was done all at once and I could avoid any further
surgery.

I already had plenty of stomach fat to spare, so decided on a
TRAM flap for my reconstruction. I was horrified to learn that
there were videos of the procedure on YouTube. Phil was fasci-
nated and, wanting to understand what I was going to endure,
watched in the name of research. I couldn't stomach them. Had I
seen even a small clip of a TRAM flap being performed I'd have
lost my nerve for sure.

My breasts weren't sexy to me; they were live sticks of dynamite
that had to go. Whatever sex appeal they'd had before I became
a mom, after nursing four babies, I couldn't see anything sexual
about them at all. They were pendulous, lopsided, and entirely utilitarian. Once I'd weaned Kivi, they'd lost their utility as far as I was
concerned. I would thank them for their service and give them an
honorable discharge before they tried to do me in.

Dr. Giannaros recommended two NYC cosmetic surgeons she
frequently worked with. I called both offices to schedule a consultation. One had only 7:30 AM time slots available. To get from
central New Jersey to the Upper East Side appointment, I'd have
had to leave my house at 6:00 AM. So, I booked a consult with
the other surgeon at a civilized 11:00 AM. And that, my friends, is
how I make important medical decisions.

A week later, I found myself standing against a bright white
wall in an exam room, stripped from the waist up, hands on my
fleshy, stretch-marked hips, belly rounded and sagging. A decade
of constantly sucking in my gut made it difficult to let it all hang
out. It truly felt more vulnerable than having four eyeballs scru-
tinize my breasts. Dr. Maitlin, a well-groomed, soft-spoken man,

sat on a wheelie stool opposite me while a medical assistant stood behind him and pointed a large digital camera at me. She clicked away while Dr. Maitlin and I discussed my cosmetic objectives.

"Have you thought about what cup size?" he asked, instructing me to turn to my right. "You look like a DD now and from what I can see," he rolled up close to me and gently prodded my doughy abdomen, "you don't have enough stomach fat for that size. We can achieve a large A, maybe a small B, but no more."

All I heard was "You're so skinny!" and I was immediately disappointed in myself for caring. Ever since high school, I'd dreamed of being able to button a crisp, white blouse over my chest and not have those unsightly gaps ruin my outfit. I'd never been much of a dieter or too concerned with my weight or size, but found my huge breasts to be inconvenient and embarrassing. They stopped me from living my best tube top/halter jumpsuit/ satin slip dress life.

"An A cup is fine, I'm not really concerned with cosmetics," I said. I dropped my arms to my sides as instructed; the camera continued to click. "I'm here to save my life. I'm not a person who gets plastic surgery, no offense." Using both hands to point at my boobs, I said, "I don't care about how they look. In fact, the smaller the better. Bet none of your other patients ever say that!"

"You will care, though," he said, smiling warmly. I liked that his eyes crinkled up. He didn't look plastic surgeon-y. "When the dread of getting cancer is gone, you'll find yourself caring about things like that."

He patiently laid out the details of the procedure, how he and Dr. Giannaros would work as a tag team. First she'd remove all my breast tissue, leaving nothing behind but empty bags of skin, and he'd step in to tunnel my stomach fat and muscle up through my abdomen and into my chest. He warned that I might lose up to 20 percent of power in my abdomen, that it might be a long time, or never, before I'd do another crunch or sit up. I didn't mind. I hated doing crunches anyway.

Finally, he got up, and before leaving, he made me this promise: "You're going to have a great result. You're going to have a Britney Spears stomach!" The hottest pop stars of the day were Taylor Swift, Rhianna, Pink, and J.Lo. Spears was in the news for her public breakdown, not her iconic style or her fitness level. I found his outdated celebrity refence endearing and although I would never have admitted it to anyone else, I was giddy with excitement at the prospect of having a stomach like Britney's.

What do you call that feeling when you want time to speed up but also stop completely? Because that's what I had. From the moment we set a date, life moved at the speed of a barrel heading toward the edge of Niagara Falls.

Despite my best efforts to keep it at bay, September and back to school were upon us. Ezra started second grade, Lea had a big year coming up in Primer where she'd learn to read, and Tani was off to nursery. Kivi, fifteen months, was still home with me and I cherished my hours with him in a way I hadn't with the other three. He'd been born smiling and now, with his little overbite and rhino-size, square teeth, was smiling still. I'd rock him to sleep on our glider each night, letting him doze on me a few minutes longer before placing him on his soft crib sheets.

September heralds in the Jewish new year (unless the High Holidays are late, in which case they spill over into October). For Rosh Hashanah, the kids brought home apple and honey projects and paper shofars they'd made with plastic mouthpieces that sounded like kazoos when blown. When they brought home slippers made of paper and staples, it meant Yom Kippur was around the corner. Each project marked the passage of time that was hurtling forward and I was powerless to stop it.

In addition to planning elaborate meals with friends and family after prayer services, holiday prep included buying new clothes and shoes for the kids, symbolizing a fresh, new year. Normally I spent weeks hunting down matching outfits for the kids to wear to shul and a new dress and hat for myself, but this year I was distracted and left it to the last minute, so their outfits didn't coordinate. And I couldn't have cared less.

Typically, the kids played in supervised groups elsewhere in the shul while I sat in the main sanctuary with my friends, but for the first time, I excused myself to a back corner where I could concentrate. I had important things to pray for and required solitude. The stakes had never felt higher.

By Yom Kippur, I was an emotional wreck. As its name suggests, the Day of Atonement is serious; it's the holiest day of the Jewish year. We don't eat, drink, or wear makeup or perfume, so the focus is entirely on praying for forgiveness of past sins and for a year filled with blessing and prosperity. To symbolize our humility before God, we don't wear leather shoes. Hence the paper slippers made in school. Yom Kippur is somber and holy enough as it is, but with less than two months to go before I'd be under the knife, my prayers took on a possessed, frenetic energy. I became one of those loud whisperers who holds the machzor right up to her face, literally burying myself in the prayer book. Usually, I'm easily distracted in shul. Now I stood, all in white, listening to the chazzan chant the words "who will live and who will die" and the ringing in my ears nearly sent me staggering over onto the red carpeted floor. *Let me live*, I thought. *Let me survive this, God. Please.*

I didn't even mind when Tani snuck into my pew and grabbed a fistful of my white skirt with his chocolatey hands. "Hi, Ma," he squeaked, a ring of chocolate around his plump pink lips before settling into the seat next to me. I kissed his wispy curls, wiped his mouth with a tissue, and turned my attention back to the words on the page.

In October, we went to Israel for Sukkot, a festival during which we eat most of our meals outside in a sukkah—a temporary hut with a bamboo roof to let in the sparkling starlit night. It was the farthest we ever traveled as a family, and of course, it was entirely Phil's idea. I'd have preferred to avoid a twelve-hour flight with four little kids and monstrous jet leg, no matter how beautiful Jerusalem was that time of year. Yet, Phil needed this rare break from work, and I knew it. And he promised to be responsible for sixteen-month-old Kivi for the duration of the flight. As much as I was dreading the journey, I reminded myself to focus on the upside: I'd have the chance to pray at the Kotel for my surgery to go well.

Miryam and Mikey traveled and stayed with us, as did Phil's youngest brother, Harrison, and Gita who was spending her gap year in the same seminary I'd attended at her age.

I'd been to the Kotel many times, watched other women shuckle and sway with closed eyes and upturned palms in supplication, kissing the shiny, lower layer stones of the Wall, worn smooth from decades of kisses and caresses and notes placed between the rocks. Their deep connection was clear, but I had struggled to feel anything at a wall. I'd always struggled to feel "something" in sacrosanct places. It was too contrived and didn't work for me. When I visit my parents' gravesites, my dominant emotion is awkwardness. It's so one-sided, talking to an engraved stone, like "Hey, there you are, let me fill you in on my life."

On this particular visit to the Kotel, I did not need to conjure any feelings. They flowed out of me, urgent and desperate. This time I closed my eyes and shuckled, trancelike; I held my siddur to my chest, my free hand balling into a fist in front of me, and moved in time to the words, enunciating every single one.

Please, God. Please let me survive this. Please let my efforts and willingness to choose this path pay off so I can give my children a chance to grow into adulthood with a mother. Please let my sisters see how much power we have to protect ourselves.

Please.

Please.

Please.

As I backed away from the Kotel, I realized I was crying.

Late one afternoon, after a morning of touring Jerusalem in the hot sun, the kids were sprawled on the living room couch watching a DVD of *Kung Fu Panda*. Other than the sound of the air conditioner on full blast, there was the quiet and tranquility that only screen time can offer. I was tidying up, collecting their sweaty socks and the morning's discarded pajamas, and paused behind the couch to watch for a few minutes. I was just in time to hear Grand Master Oogway share his prophecy with Master Shifu that Tai Long, their mortal enemy, would soon be a threat to their village again. Shifu is incredulous and splutters his protest that it is impossible. Tai Long, he reminds Oogway, is locked away in prison under round-the-clock surveillance. Master Oogway's response is a warning: "One often meets *his destiny* on the road *he takes to avoid it.*"

My stomach flipped. The air conditioner did nothing to stop the sweat pooling in my armpits. His words, originally attributed to French poet Jean de la Fontaine I would later learn, felt like a premonition about my own efforts to batten down the hatches and protect myself from danger. I tried to tell myself it was just my anxiety rearing its persistent head, that I had no reason to think the words of an animated tortoise were prophetic about my life. I hurriedly abandoned the movie and went to the kitchen. My hands shook as I prepared dinner, causing the hot oil from the pan to splatter over me as I fried schnitzel.

Was I destined—doomed—to my parents' fate no matter what I did? Was I kidding myself that I had any control over whether or not I got breast cancer? Was that damned tortoise trying to tell me something? If he was, I refused to listen. I had to do what my mother had not; I had to *try*. I was not going down without a fight.

PRESURGICAL INTAKE FORM FOR A
PREVENTATIVE MASTECTOMY

Date: August 15, 2008

Name: Gila Pfeffer (nee Reinitz)

Age: 34

Height: 5'3" (OK, 5'2¾")

Weight: RUDE

Who referred you to see us today? My ob-gyn referred me to this practice specifically, but if you're asking whose idea it was to have a prophylactic double mastectomy, that's all me. I've been wanting to do this since I first heard about it.

Have you had a psych eval? Yes, I'm fully on board with my choice and frankly would need more of a psych eval if I was prevented from having this surgery. If you think my anxiety levels can't get any higher, oh yes, the hell they can.

Are you aware of the emotional and psychological impacts of this type of procedure? Yes, I expect to come out the other side of this feeling emotionally whole and validated and psychologically strong, maybe too strong, as though I am invincible. Are you aware of implications of me *not* having this procedure?

Do you understand that this procedure is irreversible? I certainly hope so, ma'am.

What is your current bra size? DD

Will you opt for reconstruction? Yes, but less because I care about what my boobs look like and more because of the TRAM Flap reconstruction method where they take your stomach fat and muscle and repurpose them into breasts. I've given birth four times in less than six years. If anyone's due a free tummy tuck compliments of our expensive health insurance company, it's me!

What cosmetic result do you hope to achieve in undergoing this procedure? Look, you can replace my breasts with two frozen rib eye steaks, or a pomegranate and one balled up sock—I don't care, just get these two ticking time bombs off me.

Please list all operations and hospitalizations: Unless you count the dental implant surgery I had when I was thirteen, I've never had any operations, never broken any bones (*p'tooh, p'tooh, p'tooh*), and overall I'm rather risk-averse. I'm terrified at the thought of undergoing general anesthesia or having my body cut open. I've been hospitalized four times and each time I went home with a new baby.

Last menstrual period: Oh, around three weeks ago, I guess? I've got four kids under the age of six; you're lucky I can remember my own name.

Have you experienced menopause? God, no, I'm only thirty-four!

Were your ovaries removed? No, were *yours??*

How may pregnancies have you had and how may live births? Four of each! (Thank God.)

Are you taking any contraceptives at this time? Yes, NuvaRing and it's the absolute best.

Are you a BRCA gene carrier? What gave it away? Was it the chart of dead relatives in my first intake form? My obsession over having this prophylactic mastectomy? The way I hold my pen?

Anything you'd like to ask the doctor? Well, off the top of my head . . .

Will the anesthesia tube knock my teeth out?

What if I wake up in the middle of surgery?

What if I *die* in the middle of the surgery that I'm having to make sure I *don't die*??

Will you need to shave any of my body parts? If so, which ones? AND WHO WILL BE DOING THE SHAVING??

I've heard that surgeons have a radio station piped into the OR while operating; are you sure this is a good idea?

What if they sew me up and forget they left a SURGICAL TOOL in my body and I set off airport security alarms for the rest of my life and get detained when the TSA lady can't find any metal on me, even after a pat down and I miss my flight????

Anything else we should know? I'm terrified. If I try to back out of this, please stop me.

_____

Patient or Representative Signature:

_____

Date:

6

all the single ladies

It's late at night, the kids are asleep, and my surgery is in T-minus two days. Phil has been watching me "nest" the way I had at the end of each of my pregnancies, only this time I'm preparing for the unknown. My impulse to ensure our household runs smoothly without me is on steroids.

I'm bending over the open Sub-Zero freezer drawer, taking inventory of the stockpiled food. "OK, there are three lasagnas, frozen in portions so each one can be served as one dinner. I put the meatballs and schnitzel on this side, also in nightly servings," I announce, matching the frozen meals to the entries on a spreadsheet I created. There was enough food to run a two-month summer camp for at least fifteen kids. Phil is sitting behind me at the kitchen table saying "Mmhhmmm" and "Meatballs, got it" at regular intervals but when I stand up and turn around, he's tapping away on his BlackBerry.

I slam the freezer drawer shut, stomp over to Phil and block his device with my spreadsheet. "Hon, this is important, come on. I won't be able to use my arms for weeks. I'm trying to make your life easier." I huff. He rolls his eyes and rubs his temples. We both know I'm not doing this for his sake.

"I know how to feed our kids, Gi. I can see what's in the freezer with my eyes, and I'll make sure to check items off the spreadsheet as I use them. You made so much food, I can't imagine we'll run out. Plus, didn't Tamar say she was going to check in on us regularly?" Yes, my longtime best friend was organized in ways I could only dream of. She appointed herself the captain of my recovery team, so if anyone wanted to drop off food, visit me, or help with the kids, they'd have to go through her first. It was a streamlined system that gave me reassurance.

Phil pulled me in for a hug. "I know you're scared. This is a big, brave thing you're doing and I'm in awe. Really."

Scared was an understatement; I was petrified to the brink of insanity. I'd heard too many horror stories about surgeries going wrong; a news report about a woman whose teeth had been knocked out by the anesthesia tube, a friend whose aunt went in for a routine operation and died on the table. The list of things to worry about was endless. And if I *did* make it out of surgery alive, I was looking at *six* weeks of recovery time in a beat-up leather La-Z-Boy on loan from a friend. On the one hand, an enforced period of rest sounded delightful. On the other, it meant delegating child-related matters like making sure they had their favorite placemats under their bowls, checking their backpacks for school notices and homework, cutting their fingernails, and, my favorite part of the day, bed- and bath-time. Phil, his mom, Miryam, and Sandra, our cleaning lady and sometimes babysitter, would work together to keep the household running. They were perfectly competent, I knew that. It was just that they wouldn't do things exactly the way I did and that was a lot for my inner control freak to accept.

The presurgical psych eval should have asked, "Are you prepared to be completely powerless while forced to watch the people who love you perform their imperfect interpretations of your household routine? Can you bear the thought of your husband failing to enforce the teeth brushing policy stringently enough, and letting the kids track mud throughout the house instead of barking 'SHOES!' when they come in from the backyard?" Was I cool with watching my tight ship loosen while my hands were tied?

Filling the freezer meant we could avoid the aluminum pan conga line of dishes brought by friends and neighbors. It was essential that life at home stayed normal, that my kids' routines be disrupted as little as possible—and only in good ways, like Grandma coming to visit, sleepovers on a school night, or small gifts delivered by my friends to keep them distracted.

After all, if there was one thing of which my community was well aware, it was my upcoming surgery. I'd spoken about little else since the start of the school year. If you lived in Edison, New Jersey, in the fall of 2008, you knew about it, too. I told anyone who'd listen—and several people who wouldn't. I was also telling it to myself in the mirror. Once I put it out there, I wouldn't chicken out. It was the accountability I needed.

A typical conversation with a friend I ran into at the grocery store might go something like this.

Unsuspecting Person: [pushes half-full shopping cart up to mine, keeping both hands on the handlebar as if to say "I'm in a bit of a rush"] Hey, Gila! Long time no see, how are things?

Me: [about to release the Kraken even though I, too, have places to be] Oh, you know, busy with the kids and school board meetings and, actually, I'm having a preventative double mastectomy with reconstruction because, you know, I'm BRCA1 and I want to make sure I don't get cancer like my mom did. She died, you knew that, right? So did my dad. No, don't be sorry, it wasn't *your* fault ha-ha, so anyway, I found out that I can drastically reduce my chances of getting breast cancer by getting rid of these two [cue a ta-da gesture just beneath my chest while ignoring alarmed/horrified/not-sure-what-to-say look on Unsuspecting Person's face]. Basically, my breast surgeon will scoop my breast tissue out like cantaloupes and then my stomach fat and muscle will be pulled up through my mid-section [upward jerking motion from my lower abdomen to my chest] and up into the empty skin on my chest to make new boobs. Free tummy tuck and boob job after four kids, not bad right? So, what's new with *you*?

Unsuspecting Person: [already heading back down the produce aisle as fast as their cart will go and clearly making a mental note to never ask me anything ever again] Wow, that's so, uh, wow, good luck!

With each retelling of what I was about to do, I sounded more and more like the rabbi of a congregation, sermonizing on the virtues of breast cancer prevention. All that was missing was a pulpit. If I'm being honest it was also an opportunity to welcome accolades for my bravery and dedication to my health and who doesn't like a little hit of dopamine?

Reactions to my announcement were mixed.

From my sisters, I got an unequivocal thumbs-up.

Miryam (twenty-eight, no kids yet): Coolio, I mean I don't think I need to do that, but I'm here to help. Also, you're gonna have tight new boobs and a flat stomach, lucky Phil! Do you want me and Mikey to move in with you?

Rivky (twenty-four, one baby plus one on the way): Wow, Gi, I mean, wow, that's such major surgery! To be honest, I'm not really thinking about cancer, but I'm sure you've looked into it and are doing the best thing for you. I mean, I wouldn't consider doing it myself, but I totally support your decision, of course.

Gita (seventeen, a senior in high school. Not wanting to burden her, I gave her only the haziest of details. She could wait a little longer to start thinking about prevention): Good luck, Gi, let me know how I can help with the kids. (That melted my heart.)

Friends:

You're so brave.

That's something people do?

Your mom would be so proud of you.

Are you sure you need to do that?

Free boob job after nursing four kids? Nice!

I know someone who had that procedure, she was so relieved afterward.

Will Phil be grossed out by your scar-covered body? My husband would be.

I'm here to help in any way I can.

Community:

Good for you.

It makes sense given how young your parents died.

Why would you willingly mangle your body like that?

Doesn't it make more sense to wait and see?

Maybe you won't end up getting cancer and you'll have done the surgery for nothing.

Did you ask a rabbi for permission?

I did not ask our rabbi for permission. There are many instances in which we ask sheilas—questions of Jewish law brought before a trusted rabbi—about ambiguous situations, from derailed financial dealings with a friend, to how to render countertops kosher for Passover, to whether it's permissible for a sick person to eat or drink on Yom Kippur. It's common to ask medical sheilas, too. May a person agree to have a loved one taken off life support if the doctors say there's nothing more they can do? Can you take a lifesaving medicine if it contains pig gelatin? (That's always going to be a *yes*. The primary tenet of Judaism is that life should be preserved at all costs, even if it means ingesting the least kosher thing on the planet.) A prophylactic double mastectomy for someone with my risk profile could not possibly be seen as anything other than lifesaving; that was all the permission I needed—and I gave it to myself.

When it was time to tell the kids, I took a less-is-more approach. After Shabbat dinner on the Friday night before surgery, I sat on the den floor doing a giant puzzle with the older three. Kivi had already gone to sleep, and I told the others, in my best "mom talking to kids voice," I was going to be away for a few days that week because I needed an operation on my stomach to make sure I stayed healthy. I assured them they'd have Dad, Grandma, and plenty of other people looking after them while I was away. The stomach was an easier region to talk about than my chest and the part of my body that greeted them at eye level. I was relieved they had no follow-up questions.

It's a frigid November morning when the day finally arrives. Phil's mom stayed over the night before, assuring me she had everything under control. I feel a pang of jealousy that she'll be the one taking them to school later. I enter each of my kids' rooms and press soft, lingering kisses onto each of their foreheads, pausing to watch their chests rise and fall with their breaths. They can't hear my silent, steadfast promise to come home to them. They don't know they are the reason I have the will to see this through. I stand on a little wooden stepstool painted with Ezra's name to give me enough height to lean over Kivi's crib. I inhale his scent—a mix of Johnson's baby shampoo and a diaper full of pish. I could have stayed there forever.

Phil is waiting for me in the idling car. I get in and turn to check that my hospital bag is there.

"Let's go," I say quietly. It's as much a directive for Phil to drive as it is a pump-up speech for myself.

Checking in for surgery feels almost like checking into a fancy hotel if I squint hard enough and focus on the dark wood and brass accents throughout the reception area. The waiting lounge features huge windows with sweeping views of the East River. I'm handed a neatly folded pile of hospital garb and socks to change into and I head for the nearby dressing room.

In the waiting room, people sit clustered together in teams wearing uniforms that make their roles clear: regular clothes mean support/not here for surgery. Fuzzy socks, slippers, and a waffle weave robe over a hospital gown scream "patient." The robes are a nice touch, making it feel almost like a spa. The illusion is broken every time a nurse walks in and reads a name off a chart. I expect mine to be called any minute; it's 7:30 AM and I'm scheduled for 8:00. Statistically, the first time slot of the day is the best because your doctors will be fresh and alert and full of coffee, thereby less likely to forget they left a stainless-steel clamp inside your chest before sewing you up.

I do my best to remain calm by listening to *I Am . . . Sasha Fierce*, the one album I've managed to load onto my new iPod Classic. The 41:36 run-time of Beyoncé's latest songs will be more than enough to keep me entertained until I'm called into surgery. Plus, this being the iPod with a tiny screen, I can watch videos, too. Or in my case, video. I only have one loaded onto my device: "Single Ladies." What a great dance video. At home, I'd already watched it on repeat, trying to pick up some of her moves. The waiting room gives me more time to study Queen Bey and her leotard-clad, pony-like backup dancers. I can see myself on the screen, right alongside them trotting up and down a horizonless white landscape. I think I can watch that video a billion times and never get sick of it.

When a nurse comes over to quietly tell me that my doctors have been called into emergency surgery and that mine will be delayed by a couple of hours, I'm disheartened but understanding. I'm not a jerk. Of course, an emergency trumps my elective surgery. I wish the emergency patient well and send a silent prayer up to God thanking Him for not making me the emergency. Two hours pass. Then three, four, five. Phil checks with the nurse's station every half hour for updates on when I can expect to be called in.

Five hours after first taking a seat, I'm still sitting in the waiting room. I am sick of the "Single Ladies" video. I've had nothing to eat or drink since the night before, while Phil chomps on a grilled chicken sandwich he ordered from a local kosher eatery. I also want to murder twenty-four-hours-ago Gila for not having worked harder to load more songs (and videos) onto this stainless-steel rectangle of hell.

I fall asleep on Phil's shoulder. When I wake up, the look on his face tells me that there is no update.

"You smell like grilled chicken and onions," I mumble. "It's making me hungry."

"Sorry, Gi" he says. "How are you holding up?"

My head still on his shoulder, I look up at him and shake my head.

"I don't know how much more I can take," I say, deflated. It's 12:30. Tears are threatening to appear and I squeeze my eyes to stop them. If I cry, I'll fall apart. And if I fall apart, I'll lose my resolve. And if I lose my resolve there's a solid chance I'll bolt out of the hospital and keep running like I'm Forrest Gump, hospital gown and robe flapping around me. He kisses my head and hugs me tight.

"The good news," I say, sitting up again and tightening the belt on my robe, "is that I now know the entire choreography to 'Single Ladies.'" I roll my head on my neck and flip my right hand in and out to demonstrate. "Remind me to buy an off-the-shoulder black leotard when we get home."

Morning melts into afternoon and I'm starting to hallucinate about huge bowls of linguine pomodoro, hunks of baguette, and tall glasses of ice water. Names are called for begowned patients and they file out. New ones come in to take their places and I start to wonder if this is just where I live now. Maybe I'll have my mail forwarded here. Phil replies to texts from concerned friends and family on his BlackBerry.

By 2:00 PM, when someone in scrubs finally peeks her head in and says "Mrs. Pfeffer?" I'm so high-strung I nearly hit the ceiling jumping out of my seat. I grab Phil's hand and breathe in through my nose, out through my mouth as we're led through a set of double doors into the wing of the operating room. I can no longer pretend I'm in a hotel.

"I'm afraid it's only patients past this point, Mr. Pfeffer," a staff member in blue scrubs tells Phil while handing me a tissue-thin shower cap. I place it over my head, tucking in any stray hairs. Although I must look utterly ridiculous, Phil isn't laughing. Neither am I. "Mrs. Pfeffer, why don't you hand him your glasses for safe keeping, and he'll give them back to you as soon as you wake up."

"Oh, uh, can't I wear them just until I get onto the table? I usually wear contact lenses, so without these I'm blind as a bat." I really can't see more than fuzzy shapes without corrective lenses and the thought of walking, even aided, with such poor vision is enough to send me right over the edge.

"I'm sorry," she shrugs, "no outside objects that might invite contamination are allowed. Hospital rules."

I hand Phil my glasses and we grip each other in a viselike hug. Guttural sobs issue forth from deep inside me as the abject terror I've managed to keep at bay since I kissed the kids good-bye bursts out of me. Phil is crying, too. I picture him snapping his fingers and making all of this go away, magically rendering this procedure unnecessary. He prides himself on being a fixer of problems and I know his tears are a manifestation of his complete helplessness. He can't save his wife from what she has to do.

"I'll see you soon, hon." His voice is thick and small. "I love you so much. I'll be right here when you wake up."

The walk down the hall—the smell of antiseptic sharp, its fluorescent lights gleaming—to the operating room feels miles long. I look back repeatedly at the denim and wool blob that is Phil until I can no longer make out his shape.

Through the open double doors to the OR, I see a bunch of blue blobs who must be the surgical team waiting for me. I'm surprised to hear pop music playing, like we're going to hang out and have a pizza together. If they weren't all in scrubs and caps I might have mistaken it for a surprise party. As I take that last step to cross the threshold, I shiver like a trapped mouse, grateful for the "no food or drink after midnight" policy. Had I eaten, there's no doubt I'd have vomited all over the flecked linoleum floor. Just before I enter, another nurse stops me.

"Hey, doll, I'm sorry but you can't bring that in with you," she says, pointing to my hand, which is pressed flat against my thigh. Ah, yes, the OR rules.

I lift a jittery hand and held up my contraband. Pressed between my thumb and forefinger is a recent 3 x 5–inch summer-camp portrait of my four kids. They're wearing matching black T-shirts, posing in front of a thick tree trunk. Kivi was still too young for camp, so I'd brought him along to sit with his older siblings. It's my favorite shot of them.

"I'm not going . . . I can't go . . . into surgery without it," I insist through chattering teeth. Unlike my glasses, I needed my kids with me, for courage. She gives me a sly sideways smile, pries the photo from me and seals it inside a sterile Ziploc bag. "I'll slip it under your pillow," she says, putting a finger to her lips.

I climb up onto the table and sit with my legs dangling over the side, trying unsuccessfully to pretend I am anywhere but here. Dr. Giannaros strides toward me looking glamazonian despite her mask and surgical cap. Her smile reaches her eyes, as she gives my shoulder a squeeze and apologizes for the delay.

"Ready?" she asks.

I manage a tight-lipped smile and two thumbs up; if I open my mouth to speak, I will barf up the nothing I ate that day. Someone pokes around my arm for a vein and explains that the IV drip will send me off to sleep before I'm intubated for the general anesthesia. My brain swirls with those endless thoughts of the tube knocking my teeth out, incisors flying everywhere.

The last thing I see is my precious photo being tucked under the pillow on the table where I sit with my legs dangling over the side.

The last thing I hear is a voice saying, "Now lie down and count backward from ten," while the spaced-out synthesizers and clap of the intro to, I kid you not, Beyonce's "Single Ladies" plays overhead.

And the last thing I think as my head hits the pillow, counting from ten down to nine, is: "They're going to need stronger drugs than whatever this is, I'm still awa—"

I didn't even make it to seven.

When I came to, the world was out of focus. The fog of anesthesia still lingered, and I could just make out the outline of a huge fluorescent square overhead. My other senses, heightened to compensate for my poor vision, stepped in to help take stock of my environment: clinking metal, the soft crumpling of paper, murmurs, muted rubber footsteps, mingling scents of Band-Aids and sweat (mine, I think), doors whooshing open and closed.

A masked face, female, leaned toward me. "How do you feel?" she asked.

How do I feel? Elated. Light. Safe.

I tried to speak but couldn't. My throat felt like it was full of cement. Perhaps my body, unaccustomed to sleeping for more than three hours since becoming a mother, thought I was dead and started to shut down. *Speak, dammit,* I commanded my brain, and it finally got the message that I am not dead (*Hallelujah, I'm not dead!*) and powered up my control functions again.

"Great." My voice was weak, gravelly. "Was that really eight hours? It felt like less. What time is it?" I could have slept another twenty-four.

Another mask answered, "10:00 PM." I thought of poor Phil waiting for me. He must be exhausted. I, on the other hand, felt refreshed.

Stephanie had warned me not to expect much range of motion in my arms at first. She'd had hardly any. So, of course the first thing I did was attempt to lift both arms, right there on the gurney, less to test my ability and more to show this cluster of medical staff in their light blue caps and gowns that I was not their average patient. I would raise my arms higher than anyone else who'd come before me. Behold my gravity-defying act, marvel not only at my successful outmaneuvering of breast cancer but also my arms rising like a post-surgical Clara in *The Nutcracker*. I'd be canonized into hospital lore, spoken of in reverent tones as doctors and nurses demonstrated to the uninitiated with their own arms just how high mine were able to—

"*Oooowww*, why does my arm hurt so much?" My reverie broke. Considering I'd come in to have my breasts removed, it was perplexing as to why my right arm felt like it had been severed and sewn back on.

"That's normal, your arms were strapped above your head for a long time during the procedure. It shouldn't last too long. But, hey, you did great!" Dr. Giannaros removed her mask and beamed at me. Even half blind I could see the glow of her Julia Roberts smile.

"Thanks," I smiled back, "so did you." *At least I* hope *you did.*

A few minutes later, my gurney started to move, and I floated like a levitating woman in a magic act; someone was wheeling me to the recovery area. I whizzed past figures in scrubs, blurry watercolors on the walls, a teddy bear with a bandaged ear on a nurses' station desk. I couldn't wait to see Phil—literally, he had my glasses and I'd need them to see him.

"Wait a second," I craned my neck back to meet the eye of the nurse wheeling me. He stopped. "Could you please just reach under my pillow and hand me what's there?" He rooted around before placing the hermetically sealed photo in my hand. I could make out the blurry green of the lush summer trees and four peach-colored circles with mops of dark hair. It didn't matter, I knew it by heart. I blew four kisses at them, in thanks for the courage they'd given me. I dropped my wrist to my side, clutched the plastic encased portrait to my thigh, and thought of my favorite line from the novel *Anywhere but Here* by Mona Simpson. In an emotional crescendo toward the end of the book, the main character, Adele August, describes her relationship with her teenaged daughter: "She's the reason I was born." That perfectly summed up how I felt about my own brood.

Phil was waiting for me outside a tiny cubicle in the post-op area. He looked terrible.

"You're glowing! How do you look so good?" he marveled while the nurse transferred me to a bed and propped me up with pillows. He was careful to avoid the bandaging around my chest and the four drains protruding from my hips and armpits. Not that I could feel any of it. Phil bent over and kissed my forehead then handed me my glasses. They were warm as if he'd been holding on to them the whole time.

The nurse showed me how to administer more morphine by pressing a nearby button and said I'd be moved to a private room within two hours. He left the cramped space and pulled the curtain around me and Phil. Our eyes met and we grinned. He held his palm out to mine and, because I couldn't raise my hand high enough, I gave him a soft "low five." *I did it. It's done. I can't believe it's behind me, that the worst is over.*

Four hours later, I was still in my claustrophobic cubicle. But I had unlimited access to pain meds, so I didn't mind too much. Phil handed me my iPod, which I finally remembered had one more download aside from Beyoncé: It was a recording of one of my favorite authors, David Sedaris, narrating new material live at Carnegie Hall. By 2:00 AM, I finally convinced Phil to go home to the kids. "Rest up and come back tomorrow. I'll text you when they move me to a room."

I pressed play, pushed the morphine button, and dozed off to Sedaris's nasal voice telling a story about an imagined conversation between a Border Collie and a parrot.

My buzzing cell phone woke me up. The display said 7:15 AM. "Did you get a room?" Phil asked, his voice groggy.

I glanced up and saw that same stupid curtain. Fluorescent light from the nurses' station stabbed through the mesh at the top. I heard moaning from either side, presumably more post-surgical patients who'd piled in overnight. Why were there no rooms? What if I never got out of here? My panic rose, threatening to break through the morphine.

"No, hon, but I'm sure they will soon. I'm fine," I lied, not wanting to worry him. "Love you."

"So help me if you're still there when I get back later, Gi."

But I *was* still there when he arrived at noon, and so help him, indeed. Phil was a fixer, and finally this was a problem that he could fix.

My hip-to-hip abdominal stitches left me bedridden and peeing through a catheter. My neck was cramping from being in the same position for so long. The walls (curtains) felt like they were closing in on me.

The nurses, harried and overwhelmed as patients on gurneys began to fill the corridors, did their best to keep me comfortable, but avoided eye contact whenever Phil pressed them for reasons I was stuck in recovery. We were both starting to lose our minds when one nurse, disgusted by the worsening situation, let us in on a secret: A Saudi Arabian prince had come in for surgery at the last minute and took over an entire floor of the hospital with his entourage. I was too tired to be infuriated, but Phil was not.

Outside my curtain, I heard his voice, level but firm, address the poor souls at the nurse's station: "My wife has been stuck back there for close to *twenty-four hours*. I know what's going on here. I know about the prince. Get her into a private room right now or I'm calling the news stations." Next I heard a chorus of voices saying, "There's nothing we can do" and "We don't know what you're talking about" and then Phil again, presumably with his phone flipped open, "HELLO, IS THIS CBS? I'D LIKE TO SPEAK TO A REPORTER, I'M AT A PROMINENT EAST SIDE HOSPITAL WHERE PATIENTS ARE BEING DENIED—"

"OK! I'll call someone!" I heard a panicky voice interrupt. Moments later, he sidled up to my bedside, triumphant. "You're getting a room, hon. Right now."

Fifteen minutes later, I was ensconced between crisp hospital sheets in a cool room, one that seemed impossibly large compared to my previous accommodations, in the burn unit. Phil was told it was the only place in the hospital with an available bed. I wondered whether the burn unit staff had ever dealt with a mastectomy patient before, but mostly I was relieved to be alone with Phil, away from the chaos of the recovery cubicle.

"How did you get CBS's phone number so fast?" I asked, clicking my magical pain relief button.

"I didn't." Phil grinned, plopping down into a nearby armchair. "I faked it; there was no one on the other end."

"My hero," I said, batting my eyelashes and laughing. I hit the morphine button and drifted off into a pain-free sleep.

Patients in burn units are more susceptible to infection, so it was kept even more sterile than other parts of the hospital. Flower deliveries were prohibited. So were visitors, aside from immediate family, which suited me just fine. Much to my relief, Miryam offered to spend Shabbat with me. She filled the mini fridge with homemade apple kugel, grilled chicken, and salads; rubbed dry shampoo into my hair; and massaged my aching neck and shoulders. She helped me empty and measure the fluid output from my four plastic, bulbous drains that gave me a jolt of pain if I moved the wrong way.

It was Miryam who saved the day when my morphine was replaced with Oxycontin pills. They were nowhere near strong enough to manage the agony. I wailed and writhed like a wounded hyena, but they'd already given me the maximum recommended dose for someone my size.

One nurse in particular would cluck her tongue in disgust whenever we buzzed for help. She probably thought I was in for a boob job, my vanity taking up precious space in the burn unit. She was exactly the person you don't want in charge of your comfort when you're at your most vulnerable. Miryam, ever the diplomat, kept her cool while explaining what kind of surgery I'd had and why. She didn't point out that this was all in the chart at the foot of my bed. A chart the nurse clearly hadn't consulted.

"You don't know my sister," Miryam persisted, "she has a freakishly high pain threshold. If she's already screaming like this, it means she's at a level that would make most people black out." The doctors upped my dose, and my relief was immediate. The nurse's attitude softened by a degree or two and she almost smiled when she came to deliver a bunch of balloons sent by my friends. "These came with flowers but those are a hazard to *burn* patients in the *burn* unit, so we got rid of them," she scoffed, as if I'd sent them to myself. Someone in the gift shop must have been sleeping on the job—the balloons were all light blue and printed with baby bottles, pacifiers, and bubble letters that read "IT'S A BOY!"

On my third day in the hospital, I had two monumental achievements: I left my bed to attempt walking for the first time post-surgery and I used the toilet. Both were important steps in my recovery, and both were excruciating. Instead of a bathroom with a door, my room had a freestanding toilet in the corner with a curtain that pulled across. If you're picturing a floor-length curtain, stop right there. This curtain hung from a rod a few feet above the toilet and stopped halfway down. So, the toilet was visible to anyone else in the room. And anyone who sat on it (eventually me) would be on display from the waist down. This is why I was not excited when a nurse removed my catheter, which had previously meant I hadn't had to pay attention to my bladder. Before I could attempt a trip to the bathroom, however, the nurse had to be sure I could walk. She told me to grab onto her neck with both hands and ease myself to a semi-standing position. Between my raw abdominal stitches and jelly-like legs, I felt powerless. I did as I was told, unabashedly crying in pain and frustration. I didn't stop bawling as she and Miryam escorted me and my IV pole on a stooped, halting walk down the hall, back to the room, and onto that damn toilet. By the time I made my way back into bed, I felt like I'd run three marathons.

Dr. Maitlin, the cosmetic surgeon, came by to check on me and my bandages. He sat on the edge of the bed, took my hand in both of his and smiled with his warm blue eyes while going through my post-operative care instructions, which included keeping my hospital-issue sports bra stuffed with tufts of gauze to protect his handiwork. "Everything looks good! I managed to give you a small B cup size; I think you'll love how they came out once the bandages come off," he said with pride. I reminded him that I didn't care what my breasts looked like, only that they were gone. But secretly, I was excited to see them. "You did such a brave thing and look at you, you're OK!" he continued. Be very proud of yourself." It was so pure, so fatherly, so much what I needed to hear, I had to look away or I'd start crying.

Phil came to collect me late Sunday morning and just like when I'd given birth to Ezra, I was reluctant to leave the safe cocoon

of the hospital. How would I manage up the staircase to my bedroom? What if the kids ran into my abdominal stiches? What if
my drains got infected? I wished we had a Craftmatic adjustable
bed like my parents did in Staten Island instead of the old brown
recliner waiting for me at home.

As Phil pushed my wheelchair past the nurses' station, I caught
a glimpse of Grumpy, RN, who surprised me by smiling and waving. "Best of luck, my dear. May God be with you," she called out
and I nodded in thanks.

Phil wheeled me to our car the way he had after each of our
kids was born. He helped me into the passenger seat and drove
home to New Jersey slowly, like *I* was the newborn baby.

The kids were out with my in-laws when we arrived home. I
took my time crawling up the stairs, inching my way to our bedroom. When I winced in pain, Phil did, too. I'd already mapped
out this recovery plan, which would take place almost exclusively
in the peeling leather La-Z-Boy.

Painkillers

Sleep

Sleep

Physical therapy exercises to regain arm movement

Visits from the kids

Massages from a therapist/healer who made house calls

Ignoring what was going on in the rest of the house because I
    couldn't do anything about it

Daytime TV

Painkillers

Painkillers

Sleep

The recliner became my whole world, the bathroom a vacation destination I visited several times a day. I flitted in and out of consciousness, sometimes waking up to a visit from friends bearing gifts like cushiony socks with rubber treads, stacks of novels, and from Stephanie, a creamy fleece blanket with a tiny lamb's face embroidered in one corner. She had an unfair advantage when it came to choosing the perfect post-mastectomy gift. I named the blanket Lamby.

The kids swooped in and surveyed my setup, asking to climb onto the seat with me and play with the recliner lever. The risk of them hitting my sutures and sending me into an abyss of pain seemed worth it to be able to caress their pink cheeks with mine. They brought news of their days at school.

"Today, Sammy brought a turtle to school!" —Ezra

"I was the Shabbat Mommy today, and I lit pretend candles and made a bracha just like you! Also, Shira got sent home with lice." —Lea

"Morah Shaindy gave me cookies." —Tani, whose mouth was still rimmed in chocolate.

Kivi, eighteen months, worked on mimicking sounds his siblings made but we didn't really understand him. His contribution, as always, was joy, pure and unabashed.

Between my limited mobility and throbbing aches at the incision sites, there was nothing I could do in the way of household or childcare tasks. My family and friends stepped in as a village of support, so there was nothing for me to do but focus on healing.

Shortly after coming home from the mastectomy, I found a local massage therapist willing to make house calls, a middle-aged French woman with laughter lines and a wrinkled brow who told me to call her by her Hebrew name, Elisheva. Growing up in an antisemitic French town had taught her to hide her Jewish identity; even years after moving to the US, she remained cautious. As she worked the knots out of my battered body, she spoke of spiritual things, Kabbalah and destiny. I was delighted by the way her French accent altered the word "subconscious," so it sounded like she was saying "soup conscience."

"I start every day by saying zee Modeh Ani," she said, referring to a prayer of thanks to God for restoring our souls to our bodies after a night of sleep (considered in Judaism to be a mini death). As schoolchildren, we started each day by chanting the words in class, but it had been years since I'd recited them.

"You should say eet every morning and right after, list off everyzing you are thankful for. Make sure to say eet out loud." I adopted the practice immediately.

For days, I lay suspended with my head and fuzzy-socked feet at the same height, drains dangling off the sides of my chair, basking in the glow of strong pain meds and good fortune. My prayers had worked; I didn't die in surgery. In the span of a single day, I'd broken my family's cycle of early death. My kids had their mom. Phil had his wife. Our family could now dare to envision a future in which breast cancer was not inevitable; in which living past forty felt possible. *Zaidy*, I thought, *you were only half right. It turns out I have as much seichel as I have mazal.* Maybe my good fortune was due, in part, to my ability to make good decisions.

7

meeting my destiny
on the road i took to avoid it

On the last Thursday in November, I sat in the La-Z-Boy and inhaled the scent of roasting turkey, corn muffins, and pumpkin pie wafting up from the kitchen. More comforting than the familiar smells themselves was the fact that they meant Phil's mom was in the kitchen. She was an outstanding cook and she and my father-in-law were the ultimate hosts. Their Thanksgiving feasts were legendary and, since the day I met Phil, we'd spent every Thanksgiving at his parents' house. My siblings and their extended families were always welcome to join and often did. This year, however, I was in no shape to be traveling anywhere, so my mother-in-law brought the feast—everything from mains, sides, and beverages to place settings and festive table decorations—to us. Soon, we'd sit around our dining table and gorge ourselves on roasted root vegetable soup, stuffing, cranberry sauce, and a perfectly basted, golden-brown turkey—assuming I managed to make it down the stairs for the first time since arriving home five days earlier.

Phil came upstairs to share a moment of quiet as the last of the fall afternoon sunlight faded. Earlier that day, the pain had broken through my prescription medication and left me howling like a rabid animal, pounding my fists against our bathroom wall. The pain was everywhere, and it was stunning. "WHY DID I DO THIS?" I screeched while Phil did his best to steady me without disturbing my network of drain tubes. He murmured some encouraging words about how I'd already done the hard part and how much he admired my resolve while steering me, still screaming, back to my chair. He placed a red and blue capsule on my tongue, held a cup of water to my lips, and said calming words until I dozed off.

"Are you better now?" he asked, sitting on the edge of our bed and reaching out to hold my hand. Using his other hand, he unzipped my oversize hoodie—the official uniform of post-mastectomy patients—and checked the fluid levels in my drains.

"I think the worst of it's over. I'm sorry you had to deal with that." Now that the pain had subsided and the kids were occupied with Grandma, Grandpa, Uncle Adam, and Uncle Harrison downstairs, we had a moment to bask in the solitude of our bedroom and take inventory of the many things we had to be thankful for.

The cordless phone on the tray table next to me rang, breaking our reverie. "Hellooooo," I said, grinning at Phil. My pain meds were working again, we were about to eat the best food on the planet, and I'd eliminated the threat of cancer. Life was good.

"Hi, Gila, it's, uh, it's Doctor Giannaros."

"Oh, *hi*, Doctor G!" I practically sang, in response to Phil's mouthing "Who's on the phone?"

I knew I had an excellent medical team, but a call on Thanksgiving was next level service. Surely she had her own family dinner to get to, and here she was checking on little old me. I was a lucky girl, indeed.

"So, uh, I got your pathology report back and I didn't want to wait until after Thanksgiving to call."

She sounded halting. Tense.

"*OK*," I said, no longer singing. A deep unease crept through the veil of my medicated fog.

"I'm still in shock. Your pathology showed two tiny cancers in one breast." After the word "cancer" I heard nothing else. A deafening, high-pitched whine filled my ears. I thought my liquefied insides would spill out of me and coat the La-Z-Boy. Cancer? The whole point of having a *preventative* mastectomy was to *not get cancer*. I handed the phone to level-headed, data-loving Phil, who'd been staring at me, trying to decipher my facial expressions. He'd have the wherewithal to process the news.

I stared out the window at the now steel-gray sky while Phil paced the room saying "Uh-huh" at regular intervals. He held the phone in the crook of his neck while scribbling on a notepad.

"We'll call right after Thanksgiving to schedule her in. Thank you, Doctor Giannaros, happy Thanksgiving," he said before hanging up.

Schedule? What are we scheduling? The only thing on my schedule for the next month and a half is sitting in this chair while the kids come in to give me kisses and finger-painted get well cards.

He sank back onto the bed.

"Why is there a pathology? Why were they looking for anything if it was preventative surgery?" I demanded, focusing on the wrong parts of the news.

"Gi, there's always a pathology when surgery is involved. Anything that's taken out of a body has to go to a lab for

inspection. She said so before you went into the OR, remember?"
I did not.

Dr. Giannaros had been urging me to have my sentinel nodes removed since the first time we discussed my mastectomy. Those are the first lymph nodes leading from the breast to the armpit and, as their name indicates, they are the first route cancer cells take when leaving the breast in search of other organs to settle in. Removing the sentinel nodes from the armpits and determining that they are cancer free means the rest of the nodes would be clear. She'd tried several times to convince me, practically begging me, but I refused.

"My mother's arm blew up like a rescue raft, her edema was so bad," I explained, shuddering at the memory of my mom's gigantic arm resting on a pillow supported by her other hand. Edema is a common side effect of lymph node removal, especially in my mother's case who'd had many removed. Cancer had been found in nineteen of her nodes.

"I'd only be taking out one on each side, it wouldn't be like it was for your mom. The odds of you having any edema are minimal. This is what I recommend to all my patients—but of course it's your choice," my doctor pressed, but could see she wasn't getting anywhere. When I signed my presurgical forms, I checked "do not consent" to the question about removing my sentinel nodes. I was confident the removal of breast tissue would be more than enough.

It was a decision I now regretted. Had I listened to my doctor, my sentinel nodes would have been removed during my mastectomy. Now, she had to go back in and extract some from my right armpit to make sure the cancer hadn't spread beyond my breast. I was barely over the trauma of having undergone general anesthesia the first time and now I had to do it again. I had no one to blame but myself.

I motioned for Phil to help me stand up as he continued to share what Dr. Giannaros had said on the phone. "She said the cancers were tiny, the size of two capers." The look on my face told him that I didn't know what a caper looked like. He held a thumb and forefinger so close together they were almost touching.

"Based on how tiny the tumors are she's sure you'll be clear," he said, checking his notes. "Also, no one on the surgical team could believe it. You saved your own life, hon!" And with that, I broke down.

He held me and we swayed together until I ran out of tears. From downstairs we could hear the kids laughing and running around and around from the dining room, through the living room, front hallway, and back into the dining room. I dug deep to find the grit needed to put on a happy face and join our unsuspecting family. As the kids cheered "Mommy came downstairs!," Phil helped me shuffle into my seat at the candlelit table laden with a spread straight out of a movie. It was fitting for two people who were about to deliver an Oscar-worthy performance as Normal Couple Who Did Not, Mere Moments Before, Receive the Most Devastating News of Their Lives.

I went to see Dr. Giannaros after Thanksgiving for a post-op checkup, and with a simple snip of the stiches at each site, she removed all four of my drains. It was an oasis of relief in the vast desert of my misery. She hugged me and reiterated how astounded she was by my pathology report.

"The most important thing is that you understand you saved your life. Anyone who doubted your choice won't be able to do that anymore, now will they?" She was saying all the right things and none of the wrong ones like "I wish you'd listened to me about your sentinel nodes."

"After the node removal, you'll want to meet with an oncologist," she added, handing me the card of a colleague renowned in her field.

"Wait, why do I need an oncologist? Didn't you say it was contained?" I felt queasy and couldn't bring myself to say the word "cancer."

"Odds are that it was, and that we got it all out during the mastectomy. Once I do the node dissection, we will hopefully have more assurance that this is the case. But it's a good idea to speak to an oncologist anyway, since we did find cancer and she can offer good advice on how to prevent a recurrence."

Oncologist

Recurrence

Cancer

The reason I'd opted for the most drastic measure of prevention in the first place was to ensure those words never entered my orbit. How did I end up here? I trudged out into the biting December wind, not able to enjoy my new drain-free mobility as much as I would have in different circumstances. I flipped open my phone, dialed the number on the card, and booked an appointment for two weeks after surgery #2.

The next time Elisheva came, I told her about the possibility that the cancer had moved beyond my breast. I spoke in a flat, emotionless voice while she removed her coat, wool scarf, second wool scarf, and then the silk scarf she wore over her pilled sweater, a whiff of baby powder, patchouli, and a hint of sweat suddenly enveloping me. She smelled safe. Reassuring.

"What if they find something?" I was challenging her to use her higher powers to ward off any lurking evil.

"Zay weel not," she declared with confidence.

"But if they do?"

"Zay won't. Zee cancer eez out of you now."

Before that Thanksgiving phone call, I would have believed her, this person as close to the angels as Elisheva certainly was. But if God Himself had materialized in my bedroom just then and backed her up in whatever accent God has, I'd still be full of doubt.

Four weeks after forcing myself onto the operating table for a procedure I'd elected to have, I was back in the same hospital for one I didn't want. Beyoncé did not accompany me this time— no photo of my kids, either. The simple, outpatient procedure involved cutting out a chunk from my armpit and checking the sentinel as well as a few adjacent nodes, and it would take less than an hour. My recovery would be considerably easier than last time, but this was of little comfort. I was still doing my post-mastectomy physical therapy exercises, trying to regain the full range of motion in my arms. It was going well, but now I'd have to start from scratch on my right arm. Even more annoying, I'd be sent home with another surgical drain stuck in my armpit.

The first face I saw when I regained consciousness was Dr. G's and the first question I asked her was "Did you find anything in there?" She told me that a crude inspection of the removed chunk of armpit had been conducted by slicing it in half before sending it to pathology for a more thorough investigation, and found no evidence of cancer. To me, this was like cutting a large chocolate cake in half to look for a marble that had been baked inside. Not a lot of chance of finding that marble on the first slice.

"What are the odds the pathology will come back showing something?" I demanded.

"Oh, *very* low," she flashed her megawatt smile, and I tried to believe her. I wanted to feel as confident as she looked. "There's a 90 percent chance it will come back clear."

A few hours later, Phil took me home. We drove in silence, and I considered my doctor's prediction, but it was no use. I knew in my gut I'd be among the unlucky 10 percent. I knew it the way I instinctively knew my mother's fate seventeen years earlier at JFK airport. Even my abundance of mazal couldn't save me from what was coming.

The next morning, sounds of whispered giggles and rubber-gripped pajama feet padding across the floor announced an imminent and very welcome onslaught. Using my good arm as a sort of seat belt, I reached across my chest and gripped the bicep of my bad arm, holding my fresh drain and tubing close to my body.

"Gentle, guys, gentle!" I laughed as Ezra, Lea, and Tani came running into my bedroom to assess my situation. They peppered me with questions. "Are you healthy now, Mommy?"; "Did you buy us a present?"; "Can we have a chocolate milk box for breakfast?" I'd told them I needed another operation, just like the first one, to make extra-super sure I was OK. Easing out of bed, I kissed their pillow-marked cheeks, one by one, and told them that yes, I was now healthy; and no, Phil and I hadn't brought gifts. Then I sent them scrambling downstairs for some chocolate milk.

I walked down the hall to Kivi's room where Phil had just taken him out of his crib and set him down on the rug. Since I'd had Ezra, the early morning ritual of retrieving a happy, well-rested baby had been my favorite part of the day. Pausing outside their bedroom doors to hear them singing or babbling to themselves was a joy surpassed only by their ecstatic squeals as I cracked open the door to poke my head in and sing "Good moooorning!" I'd just started to regain the ability to do that after the mastectomy and was now back to square one on my right side. I crouched on the floor to hug Kivi with my good arm while I looked up and met Phil's eyes. We gave each other an upward head jerk, married shorthand for a million different messages. Today's nod meant "this sucks but we'll be OK." Our baby boy's scent of Johnson's lavender nighttime lotion and milk enveloped me in comfort, even as I made a mental note to buy him new pajamas. His pudgy feet were straining against the fluffy yellow fabric, pulled taut from his knee all the way down. My baby was getting bigger, and I just wanted to be able to lift him out of his crib before he outgrew that too, dammit.

Now that I was a seasoned expert in surgery, I knew there would be another pathology report. Dr. Giannaros had called me on Thanksgiving, so naturally I expected a similar phone call even though it was nearly Christmas Eve. By the morning of December 23, I was crawling out of my skin with nerves. I wanted to know:

What were we looking at?

How would we proceed?

Had my prediction been right that I'd be among the 10 percent whose nodes had been squeaky clean in the OR but not so much under the thousand-times magnification of a microscope?

I called Dr. Giannaros's office, but she was away with her family for Christmas, so I was passed along to her physician's assistant. What you are about to read is masterclass in how *not* to provide medical results to a patient over the phone.

"OK, so, let's see what we've got here." She narrated her actions while I sat on the edge of my bed, not breathing or blinking. "Just give me a second to pull up your record, do-do-do-do-doooooo-do-do, you're lucky you just caught me, we're about

to close up for Christmas! Big Christmas plans, Missus Pfeffer?"
she asked cheerily, the sound of her mouse clicking and papers
rustling in the background.

"Uh, not really, no," I mumbled, too nauseated with worry to
explain that I was Jewish and had forgotten that it was Christmas
Eve altogether. In fact, it was the third day of Chanukah and
much of my energy was focused on trying to make it a cheery
one for the kids. Not easy to do while waiting for life-altering
pathology results.

"Okaaaaaaayyy, so. You had a node dissection
do-do-do-do . . . [unintelligible mutterings of her reading my
case] after a double mastectomy, which revealed two tumors
on the right da-da-da-da-daaaaaa," she went on, unaware that
her space-filler sounds and singsong recap of my medical history
posed a greater threat to my life than cancer did.

Then, finally, "Great news, your pathology came back clear!
Congrats!"

Every organ in my body, every capillary and cell, each individual mitochondria unclenched. Tears of relief pooled in my lower
lids, and I silently forgave the PA her irritating personality. After
all, it wasn't her fault she was born this way, not all of us are
blessed with superior people skills.

"Hang on a second," she said, interrupting my magnanimous
thoughts. "Looks like I was reading the wrong report, can you
believe it? They *did* find cancer in your nodes, not much mind
you, 'micrometastasis' we call them, but still, you'll probably
need chemo so—" I felt the blood drain from my face and my
heart rate triple.

*Shut up. Shut up! Shutupshutupshutup you're a moron, who
does this to a fragile person? You're not my doctor, you can't tell
me I need chemo, you're just a PA, and not even a good one shut
uuuuuuupppppppp!* I hung up on her mid-sentence and sat in

stunned silence for a long time before calling Phil to deliver the upsetting news.

"Oh, Gi. I'm so sorry," he said, sounding as crushed as I felt.

We were both at the end of our emotional rope and needed backup to get through the weekend, especially since it was a special one: Shabbat Chanukah. For the sake of the kids, Phil and I went through the motions of Chanukah on each of the eight nights, lighting the menorah, frying up latkes, and giving the kids presents wrapped in festive paper, but neither of us felt like celebrating. I asked Miryam and Mikey to stay with us for Shabbat knowing they'd go a long way to create a joyful holiday atmosphere for my kids. It would also leave space for me to stew in my Level 10 anxiety while leaving them oblivious to the fact that something was off. Shielding my kids from unnecessary worry was paramount to my own well-being. It was *my* job as a parent to worry about *them*, not the other way around.

Just before sundown on Friday, the eight of us gathered around a folding table near the living room window to light the candles on several Chanukah menorahs. Ezra, Lea, and Tani each had wooden ones they'd finger-painted in school, and the rest of us lit a large silver menorah Phil and I had received as a wedding gift. We rushed through the special blessings and songs so Miryam and I could move on to lighting the Shabbat candles on time. With our palms covering our eyes, we murmured our weekly incantation to God asking for good health, long life, compassion, and blessings for our families. The skin beneath my armpit stiches throbbed and itched. I pressed my right arm closer to my rib cage, careful not to squeeze my drain.

"Good Shabbos!" Miryam and I said loudly as we turned to kiss and (carefully) hug one another. Hearing these familiar words, the kids abandoned their game in the den and scampered up to us.

"Goooooooood Shabbos!" they sang as I bent to kiss each one of their heads. *Please*, I prayed, overcome with emotion by the sight of the four of them in matching green-striped pajamas, *protect my family from whatever hell is coming my way.*

Shabbat proved, as usual, to be a balm for my worries. We enjoyed chicken soup, pot roast, and s'mores bars, compliments of Tamar. The men went to shul, and I slept while Miryam entertained the kids. In a blink, it was time for Havdalah, a weekly ceremony signaling the end of Shabbat. Afterward, we danced around the kitchen holding hands in a circle, four adults and four kids, while singing and wishing each other a good week. I guess my anxiety was a Shabbat observer, too, because as soon as the flame of the Havdalah candle was extinguished, my chest started to tighten, and my hands went cold and clammy. The peace of the day was gone and in its place was a feeling of terror that seemed to have doubled in strength. In an instant, the kitchen went from a hub of spiritual jubilation to nothing but a mess of dirty dishes, a floor covered in challah crumbs, and grubby kids in need of a bath. I had a burning urge to clean everything and everyone, but lacked the mobility or strength to do anything about it. If there's one thing control freaks don't like, it's feeling helpless.

"I'm going to give the kids baths," I announced, ushering them toward the stairs.

"Gi, I got it, just sit and relax. Mikey will help me," said Phil.

"OK, well then I'll vacuum the downstairs, it's gross," I said, clearly delusional.

"Gi, it will get done when it gets done. It's not important right now," he went on, demonstrating that he had a death wish. The demon inside me was summoned and I let it rip.

"Why does everyone here think they know better than me? I just want this house cleaned up and I want it done now and if you're not going to do it, I WILL!!" I couldn't say for sure, but I might have been foaming at the mouth, so rabid was my unwar-ranted rant. In the deep recesses of my mind, I knew I was being unreasonable and incredibly unfair to Phil. I could dump my rage on him, but he couldn't direct his at me. But I was powerless to stop myself.

Instead, he channeled his frustration into running the vacuum cleaner aggressively over the kitchen floor while glaring at me. Good, I thought, my need for control temporarily satisfied now we were both ragey. *And* I won't have to feel crumbs underfoot when I walk. Miryam and Mikey were on their way back down-stairs as I headed up to bed.

"Gi," she ventured carefully, "go easy on Phil. It's hard for him, too." I looked away, full of shame but she pulled me in for a goodnight hug. "Go to sleep. We'll go hang with Filbert." Her nickname for Phil made me laugh, as it always did.

As I closed my bedroom door, I heard a thud from downstairs, probably the vacuum banging into the baseboards, and felt guilty for driving Phil crazy. I vowed to get a grip, to do better. The next morning, on my way to the kitchen, I passed a bagel-size hole in the striped foyer wall. I didn't need to ask who'd put it there, nor who'd pushed its creator over the edge. Phil walked over and we stood side by side, considering the hole.

"I'm driving you crazy. I'm sorry, hon. I'm just really freaking out."

"I know, Gi. If I could switch places with you I would, really. But . . . I mean, can you cut me a bit of slack?" he asked, rubbing his shoulder.

"Well, at least you managed to hit the middle of a cream stripe. That'll make it easier for me to fix." I took pride in being the one who handled all home-maintenance tasks. It would be a challenge to spackle, sand, and paint the wall's crater with my compromised right arm, but it would be a good distraction.

"You're welcome," he said, and we looked at each other and laughed.

Later that morning, I threw a black cashmere poncho over my shoulders, and walked around the corner to the kids' school for their annual fundraising breakfast. The poncho was as much a sartorial choice as a means to hide my drain and wonky arm. Ponchos don't get nearly enough credit for the hard work they do turning flaws into fashion. I might have skipped the event altogether but felt duty bound as a current board member and past PTA president. Plus, I really needed to get out of the house.

While milling near the buffet of scrambled eggs, bagels, and lox, I forced a smile and the disingenuous reply, "GREAT!" to anyone who asked how I was doing. I was more forthcoming with Benjy Silverberg, a fellow school parent who was a cardiologist and the head of an emergency room at a local hospital. I shared my shocking pathology news and my frustration about having to wait until after the holidays to have my now empty drain removed. "I can help with that," he said brightly and ran home to get some medical supplies. Twenty minutes later he was at my kitchen table and with two snips of his gleaming shears, my stiches came loose, and the tube slipped out. The relief was immediate. I leaned back in my chair, but I couldn't fully relax. Later that week, I'd have my first consultation with an oncologist and the thought made my insides churn. That maddening PA's voice singing "chemo" was on a loop in my brain.

"You can call me for help any time, I'm just around the corner," Benjy offered sincerely. "How's your head?" he asked, referring to my mental state. That single question made me feel so understood and was all it took to crack my tough veneer. My head dropped into my folded arms on the table, and I sobbed.

"I figured as much," he said with such gentle compassion it made me cry even harder.

On a gray, slushy day in early January, Phil and I stepped off the elevator of another building in Manhattan and approached the reception desk. I'd woken up early that morning to wash and blow dry my hair and apply some makeup, no small feat given the limited use of my right arm. An array of clear, plastic display holders containing business cards of medical practitioners took up half the counter. All of their titles had some form of the word "oncology" in them.

We settled into seats in the waiting room, as far away as possible from the rest of the women there, nearly every one of whom wore a headscarf, floppy hat, or turban. No one wore a wig or makeup. They reminded me of my mother when she was sick. I promised myself, perhaps naively, that I'd always show up to my appointments looking like I'd made an effort and tried to ignore the possibility that these women had made similar vows when they first started treatment.

"Missus Pfeffer?" came a friendly voice from behind us. As if performing a well-rehearsed dance, Phil and I turned in unison toward the petite, young woman holding a clipboard in the doorway to the examining suite. "I'm Tara Seagle, you can come with me." She wore cheery red lipstick, her hair cut into a jet-black bob, and smiled just the right amount for someone who wanted to project warmth but was also about to upend my world. Under all of that though, I am not exaggerating when I say she looked fifteen. While gathering our belongings, Phil and I exchanged surreptitious raised eyebrows at each other and followed the female Doogie Howser into a small consultation room. Dr. Seagle gestured to two upholstered seats and sat behind her desk to face us. A framed photo of a little boy, maybe three years old, playing with a blue toy truck told me that she was a young mom, just like me. As she sat down, I noticed a slight protrusion in the front of her lab coat. She was pregnant.

"I just had a look at your notes," she said, turning her attention to the computer screen, "and I've never seen a case like this before. You know you saved your own life, right?" I did, as a matter of fact, but never tired of hearing it. I just wished I'd managed to save my own life while also *not* needing an oncologist.

"Given your young age, family history, and genetic profile," she went on, "I recommend a three-tier approach to your treatment. Chemotherapy, followed by hormone therapy—in your case, having your ovaries removed to stop any estrogen production, and when that's done, five years on Arimidex. It's a daily pill which blocks any residual estrogen." While the chemo would stop my period initially, the oophorectomy would put me into permanent menopause. I didn't mind going into menopause at thirty-five; I was done having kids anyway and whatever the symptoms were, I'd manage them. However, I very much minded the chemo part of the plan. I'd seen its effects up close and was desperate to avoid them.

"The standard chemo for your type of cancer—estrogen positive/Her2 negative—is a regimen known as ACT. Four doses of Adriamycin with Cyclophosphamide and then four doses of Taxol over the course of sixteen weeks." The drug names sounded alien and ominous. I squeezed Phil's hand so tight it turned purple.

Then I pushed back on the chemo.

"But didn't we get all of the cancer out in the mastectomy and the node dissection? Why do I need chemo?" My voice wobbled while I held back tears. And some throw-up.

"Technically, yes, and you only had micrometastases in two nodes. One of the nodes," she consulted her screen before turning back to me, "showed only six cancerous cells. The chemo would be a precaution, just to make sure there are no traces left." It sounded like killing an ant by dropping an anvil on it.

"So, what if I decide to skip the chemo?" I caught Phil's pleading look out of the corner of my eye.

"You could walk out of my office right now, never come back and, in all likelihood, you'd be fine," said Doogie Howser, MD, the kindness in her deep-set hazel eyes leveling me. My temptation to flee was visceral. "But I don't recommend it."

"Gi . . ." Phil warned. He knew I was considering my options, but as he saw it, there was only one: do anything necessary to ensure my survival.

"OK, but is there anything that won't make me lose my hair?" Phil let out a sharp breath of relief.

"Unfortunately, ACT has a 100 percent rate of hair loss. I'm so sorry," she said as I grimaced. "It's a major inconvenience, I know." Getting stuck in bumper-to-bumper traffic while finishing the last sips of a twenty-four-ounce iced coffee was *inconvenient*. Several alternative words came to mind as she listed some common side effects of my treatment.

Hair loss—*all* hair. Yes, *there, too.*

Mouth sores

No menstruation

Neuropathy—a numbness in the hands and feet so I'd have the fine motor skills of a toddler

A green-hued complexion—useful if I decided to audition for the role of Elphaba in *Wicked*

"I recommend you buy a wig before you start treatment," she said, scribbling something on a prescription pad. A fancy one." I saw myself pushing a grocery cart through Stop & Shop with a

Marie Antoinette-style wig festooned with satin bows towering above the produce displays while I yelled about cake. What she meant, though, was that I treat myself to a good quality, natural-looking wig.

She tore the prescription from the pad and handed it to me. CRANIAL PROSTHESIS it said, in all caps. It made me want to laugh and cry at the same time.

Dr. Seagle turned to Phil. "Any questions I can answer for you?"

He had a few.

"We're planning to move the family to London for my job this August. Can we still go?"

"Absolutely," she said without hesitation. "Gila will have finished her treatment by then."

"What about sex?" he asked, and I turned to him bug-eyed. *What about it?? Weren't you listening to all of the side effects I'm going to have? I'll be a total goblin; you want to have goblin sex?? I don't think so!*

But then I considered the subtext of his question. He was asking: How else will life as we know it be upended? How will all of this impact our marriage of only nine years?

Shifting her gaze back and forth between us, my doctor took her time and was selective with her words.

"Well, you have to be careful. The chemotherapy can potentially be passed along through body fluids, so it's best to use extra protection."

"You mean I can pass my chemo to him?" I asked, horrified at first, then thought, *Good, then we'll both be bald.*

"I guess what I'm saying is," and here she paused and took a deep breath, "you don't want to be sticking things where they don't belong." Her reply was earnest and therefore unintentionally hilarious. I avoided Phil's gaze and knew he was avoiding

mine; one look and we'd both be in the throes of an uncontrolla-
ble giggling fit.

On our way out, Dr. Seagle handed me a stack of pamphlets.
One had a list of chemo-adjacent prescriptions I needed to order,
including an anti-nausea pill and syringes of Neulasta, injections
to keep my white blood cell count up and reduce my risk of
infection. Another contained information about protocols while
undergoing treatment. On the cover, there was a photo of a smiling woman, clearly bald under her blue headscarf. We set a date
for my first infusion—January 27—and agreed that in the interim
period, a trip to Miami with my kids and mother-in-law would be
good for my mental health.

"See you back here in a few weeks!" I said brightly, as though
Dr. Seagle and I were friends rather than doctor and patient. I
stole another look at her pregnant belly as Phil and I left her
office. She was so vibrant and literally full of life; I'd soon be full
of toxic chemicals.

If you have some post-surgical healing to do and also need to
psych yourself up for four months of grueling chemotherapy,
what better place to do it than your in-laws' ocean view apartment on a Miami beachfront? They'd bought the place a few
years earlier to get away from the New Jersey winters and now it
would allow me to escape my reality for a short while.

A few days after meeting Dr. Seagle, I flew down to Miami with
assistance from my mother-in-law and Gita, who'd interrupted
her gap year in Jerusalem to help me. I'd been cleared to fully
immerse myself in water by then and reveled in the weightlessness
of floating in the apartment building's pool. The scenes around
me were a balm to my frazzled psyche: Tani, three, asleep on Gita
while she gently bobbed in the water, and Ezra and Lea, seven
and five, doing messy art projects with Grandma while eating ice

pops under the poolside gazebo. Kivi, nineteen months, rode with me. I pulled him behind me in a yellow inflatable tube while he giggled and splashed with his pudgy hands. I did my best to turn my eyes into a camera, taking mental snapshots and storing them to draw on for comfort in the terrible months ahead.

I stared at the palm trees overhead and, *CLICK*, committed them to memory.

Lea licking a river of red sugar sliding down her arm: *CLICK*.

The turquoise water of the pool lapping over the tiled edge, a flock of seagulls flying overhead to the nearby beach: *CLICK, CLICK, CLICK*.

I tilted my head back into the water and came up with slick, soaking wet hair, something I rarely did in my lifelong battle against my God-given frizzy curls. I closed my eyes and willed the sensation of cool, slippery pool-hair to imprint onto my memory.

8

cranial prosthesis

"Trust me, once you start wearing this wig, it'll make you feel so sexy you'll never want to take it off!" said Tova, my Jewish wigmaker, as she held a wheel of hair samples next to my head. We were trying to match my natural color.

"No," I said through a weary half smile, "I won't."

I wouldn't have even been in Tova's wig salon, or any other for that matter, if it wasn't for Phil's brother, Adam. I'd have been in the drugstore scanning the wall of novelty head toppers behind the register, aiming to choose one based on two criteria alone.

1. Closest match to my natural hair color

2. Least flammable

Adam is younger than Phil by four years and both of them are lawyers. Unlike his older brother who opted to work for a large

NYC firm, Adam joined their father's boutique firm in New Jersey. Phil and Adam look so much alike, people often confuse the two. At my engagement party, someone handed me a thirty-six-dollar check as a gift; it was made out to Gila and *Adam*. He's still waiting for me to give him his eighteen dollars. Whenever Uncle Adam came to stay with us for Shabbat, he brought shopping bags full of gifts and would drip-feed them to the kids every hour. He came so well stocked that each time he left after the weekend, there were still several unopened toys.

A few days after Dr. Seagle handed me the cranial prosthesis prescription, Adam called me. "I have a friend who's also a client. Her name is Tova, and she makes really high-quality wigs. I told her you're coming into the shop and to give you whatever you want. Don't ask about prices, it's all taken care of."

I'd been on the receiving end of so much kindness and support already, but this was at another level. It was the help I didn't even realize I needed. Tears pricked the corners of my eyes.

"Adam, I can't let you pay for a wig, those things cost a fortune—" but he cut me off, saying he wouldn't be paying. Sometimes their small business clients bartered their goods for his services, and he'd count the value of the wigs toward their outstanding invoices. He'd discussed the trade with my father-in-law who agreed wholeheartedly. I was more than a little tempted by this prospect of maintaining a shred of dignity, something a drugstore wig couldn't offer.

"But that's the same as you paying for them. It's too much for something I'll only wear for a year." Custom human hair wigs went for upward of five thousand dollars.

"Gila. Stop. You're going. Here's her number, she's expecting you."

I'm sure I made him—a single guy not yet thirty, sitting behind a mahogany desk in a suit and tie—deeply uncomfortable with my wet, blubbery sobs of gratitude. There's a saying in the Talmud that translates to "Say little and do much." That was Adam in a nutshell.

And so, I found myself sitting in a white leather swivel chair, facing a mirror in the back room of Tova's, in Lakewood, New Jersey. I'd never been to a wig maker before. It looked more or less as I imagined with floor-to-ceiling shelves brimming with glamorous tresses secured to faceless white Styrofoam heads, and married women of all ages, their heads covered with scarves or beanies, chatting with each other while they waited to collect their orders. It is customary for Orthodox Jewish women to cover their hair once married. Brides choosing to uphold this custom will order a bespoke wig (or two) as part of their wedding prep. Often, the end result is a head of "hair" that's thicker and more vibrant than the wearer's own, an idealized version of reality. As appealing as it may sound to resemble one of Bravo's Real Housewives, I decided not to cover my hair when I got married. I grew up in a strictly kosher, Shabbat-observant home with a mother who didn't cover her hair. By the time she started covering her head, it was for illness-related reasons rather than religious ones. Around the house, she kept her bald head exposed, but when she ventured out, she wore a poufy, human hair wig on loan from a religious friend who had a spare. It made her look less like herself than when she wore nothing at all. Now here I was, taking on an identity that wasn't mine, following in her footsteps yet again.

I was furious at the indignity of hair loss. It was the most public side effect and would leave me with limited control over my appearance. No matter how natural my hair pieces turned out, there would always be something a little "wiggy" about them. Private suffering would not be an option and that drove me bananas. Unlike others who visited Tova's for reality TV–worthy mermaid tresses, I wanted only to look like myself. Hair loss would make it so much harder to hide what was happening from my kids. My whole brand as a mom was to shield and protect them from unnecessary pain and stress.

I walked out of Tova's with a receipt for two human-hair custom pieces: a shoulder-length wig with layered bangs and a "hat fall," which was made with a mesh scalp, hair starting just above the line where a hat brim would sit. I paid zero of their combined eight-thousand-dollar retail value.

"Come back in two weeks," Tova said as she walked me to the front door. "I'll cut and style them on your head, so we get the exact look you want." But the only look I wanted was the one I already had. The one that was about to be ripped away from me.

While hair loss (100 percent guaranteed!) is the best known and most conspicuous side effect of chemotherapy, there are plenty of other serious reactions the body can have. My first chemo appointment was set for the end of January, only a few weeks away and some preparation was required. In addition to getting a (fancy) wig, I had to fill a prescription for Emend, a strong anti-nausea pill. The yellow pills in the blister pack were the largest I'd ever seen and, ironically, just looking at them made me nauseous. I also needed to have a dose of Neulasta ready and waiting in my refrigerator, a white blood cell booster, administered by injection at home about twenty-four hours after each infusion. Finally, I needed a steroid to ensure my body didn't have a violent allergic reaction to the poison being pushed into it. And all of that was before I tried to *mentally* prepare myself for my entry into what I could only envision as the fiery pits of hell.

Until that point, I hadn't taken much more than Advil, Tylenol, and the occasional course of antibiotics. I was alarmed by how medicalized my life had become. The sight of so many prescription boxes lined up on my kitchen counter the day before my first chemo treatment filled me with rage. Every other Monday, a single syringe of Neulasta arrived by courier in a white, Styrofoam box (distant relatives, perhaps, of those heads in the wig shop) and packed in ice. At three thousand dollars a pop—the amount billed to my insurance for each dose—such protective delivery measures made sense. I put my best friend Tamar in charge of administering the shot to me, so one of her many jobs was to come by my house a day after each of my infusions and watch me pull my sweatpants halfway down so she could jab my butt. I liked to stress her out by jerking to one side and shouting, "Don't drop it or you'll have to pay for it ha-ha-ha-ha!" which she never found as funny as I did.

Here's a piece of advice: DO NOT read the thick leaflet of information printed in a three-point font that comes with prescriptions and lists all possible side effects, no matter how unlikely. For Emend, these included headaches, stomachaches, a wide variety of rashes, and vomit resembling coffee grounds. Let me say that again: POSSIBLE SIDE EFFECTS OF THIS ANTI-NAUSEA MEDICATION INCLUDE VOMITING COFFEE GROUNDS.

It was enough to send me over the edge. I bawled into the phone as one of the nurses in my oncologist's office tried to calm me down by saying that in her twenty-plus years in the field, the coffee-barf thing had happened to zero of her patients.

On the morning of January 27, 2009, I stuffed three books, a newspaper, and a selection of snacks into an oversize tote bag while the kids finished their bowls of Cheerios before school. How many Nature Valley Honey & Oat granola bars were sufficient for an eight-hour session in a chemo chair? Six? I threw in a seventh just in case, nestling it next to a Ziploc filled with apple slices, a plastic container of leftover lasagna, a bag of almonds, and four twelve-ounce bottles of Poland Spring water. The Very Hungry Caterpillar Goes to Chemo.

"Where ya going, Ma?" Ezra asked with his mouth full.

"Oh, I'm meeting a friend in New York, and we've got a, uh, big day!" My voice was so artificially bright, I could have been a Nickelodeon TV show host.

"Mama!" Kivi grinned from his high chair. I picked two Cheerios off his cheek and gave him a million kisses while he giggled and patted my face with his pillowy baby hands. I could feel their sticky residue cling to my skin when I finally pulled away and resisted the urge to wipe it off.

"OK guys, backpacks and coats, time for school!"

I'm a normal mom doing normal things, you kids have nothing to worry about, I will stop at nothing to protect you from unnecessary trauma, tra-lee-la-lee-laaaaaaa.

I'd been blessed with kids who noticed only what was in their direct line of vision and were satisfied with surface level information on anything that didn't pertain to them. Also, I was a pretty decent actress, a critical skill when you're trying to keep your cancer treatment hidden. When I told the kids about my preventative mastectomy, I simply said I was having surgery on my stomach (true) to stay healthy (also true). They didn't have any follow-up questions other than "Can we watch extra TV while you're in the hospital?" The node dissection was an outpatient procedure and barely interrupted my mothering duties. I saw no point in rocking their worlds with information they didn't need. My way of dealing with this "inconvenience," as Dr. Seagle had put it, was to shield my kids and in that, shield myself from having to carry their anxieties. I had enough of my own to hold. Maintaining normalcy at home would take a lot of energy and planning but it would also be a welcome distraction. I'd be like a character actor throwing herself into a role. The biggest challenge would come when my hair eventually started falling out. That would make it incredibly hard to keep up my charade, but I told myself I'd figure something out when the time came.

Phil and I spent the forty-five-minute drive mostly lost in our own thoughts and in the pop music drifting from the radio. We held hands on and off and, when we did speak, kept our chat on mundane topics like how high the plowed snow was piled along the road or the brightness of the winter sun.

We pulled up to the building on East 68th Street and sat quietly for a few minutes, my head on Phil's shoulder while Rihanna belted "Just live your life . . . A-ay-a-ay-a-aayyyyyyyy." *I'm trying to, RiRi. Why else would I be here?*

"Are you sure I can't come up with you?" he asked as I unbuckled my seat belt and opened the door. "I can take the day off, no problem." He was pushing himself beyond his comfort zone for me and I loved him all the more for it. He had shouldered so much already, but the chemo suite was no place for him. In crisis mode, there was no one better than Phil to have by your side. If it wasn't for him, I'd probably still be in that post-surgical recovery cubicle waiting to be moved to my own room. But to sit by helplessly and watch me suffer for hours on end? That would drive him insane, which would, in turn, drive *me* insane. Plus, I was adamant about going to my first round of chemo alone, like a hero's journey.

"Hayley is on duty today," I reassured him. "She'll pick me up when I'm done, and I'll text you when I get home. I love you, hon." I kissed him goodbye and tried to look confident as I walked away from the car.

Hayley was one of two close friends I allowed to sit with me during treatments. The other was Effy who was Phil's good friend, too. I kept such tight control over who I let into the chemo suite with me, you'd have had an easier time gaining access to the Federal Reserve Bank. Not even Tamar was granted access, even though she'd have done a fine job looking after me. There was no logic behind this other than my desperate need for autonomy. Tamar, being the excellent friend she is, didn't push back.

I met Hayley, a Londoner, during my gap year in Israel. She was the only British person on the program and therefore the only other girl besides me who'd not only heard of Monty Python, but could quote verbatim from *The Meaning of Life* and *Life of Brian*, two of the funniest movies I'd ever seen. It was friendship at first quote. Eventually we landed in the same New Jersey community and had kids who became friends.

Effy grew up in the suburb we now called home and, like me and Phil, had four young kids. He and I bonded over our sense of community obligation while sitting on our kids' school board, which was only bearable since we could laugh together at what a waste of time those meetings were. Effy, Hayley, and I lived within blocks of each other and sent our kids to the same Jewish day school.

Plenty of offers came in from other friends and acquaintances to drive me to and from my appointments and sit with me for hours while the chemicals drip, drip, dripped into my veins. Everyone wanted to help, to feel useful, and maybe to express gratitude for not being the one in the shitstorm by doing a good deed. I had exactly enough bandwidth to manage the physical and emotional toll of my ongoing medical saga while maintaining household homeostasis for my kids. I didn't have a shred more to give. The tighter I kept my circle, the easier it would be to compartmentalize what I was dealing with, to pretend I was still my old self and not have repeated conversations about "how I was doing." I wasn't keeping people at bay to be cruel or exclusive. I was protecting my already teetering mental stability. If you ever find yourself at the center of a crisis, the best piece of advice I can offer is this: *You* call the shots according to *your* own needs. If anyone gets offended by not being granted a better seat to your shit show, well that's their problem.

I sauntered into Dr. Seagle's office wearing my standard uniform: a black merino wool turtleneck, denim skirt, and black leather boots which I hoped would convey "peer" rather than "patient" to my pregnant oncologist. I was already envisioning a future where we'd meet up for coffee and talk about friend things; the doctor/patient era of our relationship would be but a blip on our radar screen. Before my infusion, she had to take my vitals and wrote the order for my chemotherapy mixture to be prepared. I had to follow that same protocol for the rest of my treatment, which would take place once every two weeks. In those final moments before starting what would be my first dose of eight, I felt protected sitting across from her desk while she conducted this last bit of admin. My body was still a chemo virgin. The last time I sat here, squeezing Phil's hand while Dr. Seagle laid out my treatment plan, I'd wanted to bolt. Now, I wanted to avoid what was coming next by staying in her office forever.

Reluctantly, I followed a nurse to the chemo suite, where I kept my eyes straight ahead as we picked our way past a row of women in recliners, their drips already in progress. I didn't want to see them. I didn't want to identify with them. In my peripheral vision, I saw that every patient had someone with her, and I was proud of my choice—a little smug, even—to go it alone. I was also stupidly pleased with myself for looking so vibrant and well with my shiny hair and peachy complexion marching past the chemo chorus line to the very last seat against a wall.

It took fifteen minutes to set up fluid bags, clear tubes, and an IV pole. I was sitting upright in a pink pleather recliner, close to the

edge so as to avoid unnecessary contact with hospital furniture.
I knew that every surface there was wiped down with antiseptic and was probably cleaner than my own home, but as a germaphobe with an overactive imagination, the thought of having
to make contact with a chair that surely held the sweat, tears,
and hair of countless others nauseated me almost as much as the
thought of having chemo. I made a mental note to bring a bed-
sheet from home next time.

"Would you like a blanket?" the nurse offered.

"No, thanks," I smiled politely.

Blankets are for sick, shivering chemo people and no, I don't
want your magazines or fuzzy hospital socks or anything else to
bring my awareness to my present surroundings. I didn't even
want an ice cap, a torturous and unreliable method of slowing
hair loss by wearing a frozen helmet during infusions. From what
I'd read, ice caps had a low success rate. I wanted to be left alone
to sit for eight hours while organizing my purse and updating my
contacts in a spiral-bound address book. No, I would not like to
lean my (germtastic) chair back. Please go away.

"I'm all good, thanks," I said when she finally ran out of things
to offer me from the chemo suite menu.

As she left, another nurse approached and said, "Hello, I'm
Rose." She wore two surgical masks and a clear face shield. And
gloves. And a plastic apron over a yellow disposable gown, two
layers of cover over her scrubs. I wore no protective gear at all.
I felt exposed. She tied a rubber tourniquet around my arm and
tapped until she found a nice juicy vein into which she could
thread an intravenous needle. "First, I'll flush out your veins with
saline solution and then I'll attach your IV to the AC," she said,
pointing over my shoulder at a clear plastic bag filled with what
looked like red fruit punch. A label on the bag was printed with
"Adriamycin and Cytoxan" in sinister block letters. I felt sick

and I wasn't even hooked up to the drip yet. "Don't be surprised when you go to the bathroom and your urine is red just like that liquid," she warned without cushioning the blow. I already didn't like her.

"OK," I said, as she slowly got to work connecting the tube dangling from the pouch to the cannula sticking out of my left arm, the whole time muttering, "Yes, careful now, that's it," under her breath. It did not inspire confidence.

"Why are you wearing so many protective layers?" I asked, partially out of genuine concern, but just as much to drown out her anxiety-inducing pep talk. I could see the fruit punch moving through the tube toward my vein at a glacial pace. It was like a torture method from a movie where the antagonist dangles the hero over a tank full of angry sharks, lowering him bit by bit. Unlike in the movies, no one was going to swoop in from the paneled ceiling overhead to rescue me.

Rose jerked her head up and glared.

"This is *very* dangerous medicine I'm working with here, ma'am!" she spoke in a breathy, reverent tone. "It can be deadly! I can't risk getting even a *single* drop on my skin, it could burn right down to my bone!" I made a mental note to request that she never administer my drugs again.

With my line firmly in place, she left me to marinate in my own terror. I stared out the window at the Hudson River, trying to get my heart rate back to normal before reaching for my address book and getting to work updating names, phone numbers, and birthdays. I did my best to keep the IV pole and its tubing out of my line of vision as the scarlet river snaked down the tube toward my arm. I had no appetite and no use for the buffet in my tote bag.

About two hours in, I really needed to pee, but was loath to leave my corner office. I didn't want to walk past the other women or be exposed to the sights of my new world. Behind my eyelids, I summoned the palm trees of Miami, the choppy ocean waves, but my bladder was relentless. I grabbed hold of my tethered IV pole and dragged it to the bathroom, taking care to not dislodge the clear tubing lest it spray my red poison at everyone in its path (preferably nurse Rose) like an out-of-control fire hose.

In the bathroom, I calculated how much longer it would be until I was done, and Hayley could come take me home. I got lost in my thoughts about what my kids might be doing at that moment when I went to flush the toilet and gasped. Staring back at me was a bowl full of red fruit punch. I was halfway to fainting before realizing it was the Adriamycin. Shaking uncontrollably, I tried to calm myself with long deep breaths and sharp exhalations. It didn't work. Half-dizzy, my pole and I made our wobbly way back to the end of the chemo suite, but this time I forgot to not look at the other patients. Finally, I glimpsed my future. Wool beanies with no hair peeking out, silk scarves tied tightly to bald skulls, green/gray complexions with sunken, eyebrow-less eyes and, worst of all, blankets up to their chins.

The combined effect of my bathroom scare and seeing the bald-faced (sorry) truth of what was coming for me was my undoing. My tears came hot and fast, and I scurried back to my seat where I finally lost it, sobbing loudly into my coat draped over the arm of the chair. Coming here alone was a bad idea.

A nurse (not Rose), middle aged and wearing a colorful headband in her short, black hair, appeared out of nowhere and took my hand—the one without a cannula in it—and massaged it in an effort to calm me.

"My dear," she began in a strong Trinidadian accent, "Shhhhhhhh, it is OK, sshhhhhhh." I kept on wailing, cursing myself for telling Hayley not to come until my infusion was finished. What a fool I was to think I was above needing support.

The nurse must have assumed that my tears were due to a poor prognosis, that like countless other patients who'd been in her care, my life was on the line because the next thing she said was, "Make plaaaans for da future," waving her free hand in a dramatic arc, which made me think of Sebastian the crab from Disney's *The Little Mermaid*. I was powerless to stop my brain from picturing the nurse standing before an oceanic backdrop in a crab costume, singing a song about my plight.

"Chemotherapy" (to the tune of "Under the Sea")

So, you got a gene mutation
I think it called "BRCA1"
Well now start your celebration
You in for eight rounds of fun

You should make plans for the future
Could have had a worser fate
If you caught your cancer later
You'd be at the pearly gates
Whoa-ooh

Chemotherapy . . .
Chemotherapeeeeeeee
Darling it sucks here
Soon you'll have no hair
Take it from meeeeeeee
Now wait for nausea to set in
And mouth sores make it hard to grin
Hide in your lair now
You with no hair now
Chemotherapeeeeeeee

I grabbed my phone from the tray table and dialed Hayley's number. She picked up on the first ring.

"How fast can you get here?" I gurgled, my voice thick and nasal.

"I've been sitting in my parked car around the corner for the past two hours. I'll be there in five."

I swear I could hear angels singing hallelujah as she ran toward my chair.

"So damn stubborn, you are, Bwian," she tutted, using the Monty Python nickname we'd called each other since we were eighteen. We cackled like hyenas, fully aware of the stares from my fellow suite mates. I now understood why none of them was there alone.

Eight hours after I crossed the threshold of the chemo ward, it felt like eight years had passed. I was spent, like I'd run three consecutive marathons. Hayley propped me up with her shoulder as we walked toward the elevator. Nurse Sebastian came running after us and thrust a thick, hardback book into my hands.

"It's a cookbook for you, full of good recipes to fight cancer!" she said, beaming.

I didn't have cancer. My chemo was preventative. And I didn't need a cancer-fighting cookbook.

Once the elevator doors closed, I rolled my eyes at Hayley. She read my thoughts and grabbed the book out of my hand. When we reached the lobby, without breaking our stride, she unceremoniously dumped it in the trash on our way out into the cold evening air.

Back at home, I snuck past the kitchen where the kids were being fed dinner by my mother-in-law, and crawled upstairs, peeling off my contaminated clothes and dumping them in the hamper on my way into bed. Phil called from work to check on me. "One down, seven to go. Gi. You've got this."

I closed my eyes and didn't open them again until morning.

I woke up feeling decimated but relieved that I now had a two-week reprieve until my next infusion. The first thing I did was whisper the Modeh Ani prayer, itemizing what I was most thankful for: Phil, who must have gone downstairs to give the kids breakfast, my four children, top-quality friends, and central heating that worked. The second thing I did was tug at my hair. It was still anchored to my head. I added "hair" to my gratitude list. I was not thankful, however, for how thoroughly crappy I felt. It was like someone had removed my innards and replaced them with the stuff that floats around a lava lamp. I was dizzy and crampy, but on the plus side, I wasn't nauseous. No vomiting into a plastic bowl like I'd seen my mother do too many times. I prayed it would remain that way.

Ezra, Lea, and Tani burst through my bedroom door singing "Snow day, snow day, no school today!" and Kivi trailed behind them babbling nonsensical words in the same tune, even though he wasn't yet in school.

"Are you sure?" I asked, propping myself up with pillows and craning my neck to look out the window. Tree branches drooped under the weight of what looked like at least six inches of snow.

"They're sure," Phil said, following them into our room. "School just called."

"Can we make a snowman, Mommy? And can we have hot cocoa?" The kids were jumping up and down, clapping at their good fortune. I was happy to see their smiling faces gathered at my bedside, but the last thing I needed was all of them home today. The second to last thing I needed was the start of my period, but that's exactly what I felt coming right then.

A snow day and my period on the first day after chemo. Fantastic. Dr. Seagle had warned that chemo would make my period stop but, like my hair falling out, it looked like that would take some time.

"Want me to stay home today?" Phil offered, even though I knew he had mountains of work to do. He was thirty-three and on track to make partner at his law firm soon, a goal he'd been working tirelessly toward for eight years. Our longtime cleaning lady would be in soon to help, and I had enough friends I could call for backup. I blew him a kiss from the bed and sent him on his way.

But before I could reach out to anyone, my cell phone rang. It was Hayley. "I'll be over in twenty minutes to pick up Ez, Lee Lee, and Tani, and then bring them home after they've had dinner," she declared.

She didn't ask. She had a house full of her own kids, too. She simply anticipated my needs and showed up without making a big deal of it.

Tamar came over later that day to drop off chicken and rice for dinner and to administer my Neulasta shot.

"Assume the position," she said, holding the syringe up to the light and flicking it lightly with her finger for no other reason than to make me laugh. I pulled my pajama bottoms and underwear down slightly on one side, exposing my fleshy hip while leaning over my bed. Tamar was five foot eleven inches to my five foot three inches and she had to crouch way down to plunge the needle in, which she did skillfully. It was an oddly tender moment with my friend of more than twenty-five years and one I'd come to look forward to every other Wednesday.

When Hayley dropped the older three kids off later that night, their arms were full of arts and crafts they'd made. They were wearing pajamas I didn't recognize instead of the snow gear I'd sent them out in that morning. "What a great day we had!" Hayley sang as they ran past us and into the den. "They're fed, they're bathed, they're happy. I'll get their clothes back to you tomorrow when they're out of the wash. Night night, Bwian," she chirped and left me laughing at the door.

Two days before my second chemo appointment, we took a family outing to Asbury Park to visit Adam. He lived in a beautiful, light-filled bachelor pad overlooking the beach and was always ready for guests with a pantry full of Oreos and Pringles and a fridge stocked with Diet Snapple. Phil's parents and younger brother Harrison would be there, too, our first gathering since I started treatment a week and a half earlier. The effects of my first infusion had completely worn off after a couple of days, so I felt great.

It was windy but unseasonably warm for early February and after parking the car, I suggested (demanded) that Phil and I take some family photos on the nearby boardwalk before going inside. The kids were dressed in matching chocolate-brown quilted jackets and, like Phil, wore blue jeans. They looked adorable and I looked healthy, and I had an urgent need to capture this moment of normalcy in the midst of my own personal chaos. I lived for pictures of my kids in matching outfits and knew the day would come when they'd refuse to dress like their siblings.

I handed my digital camera to a willing passerby, and she patiently waited for us to arrange ourselves across a wooden bench, me in the middle, Tani and Ezra next to me, their legs dangling, Lea on my lap, and little Kivi squirming in an effort to break free from Phil's grasp. The woman snapped away while I pointed at the camera, trying to get everyone to smile and face the same direction until they'd all had enough and started hopping down from the bench. I retrieved my camera and threw it in my bag without bothering to scroll through the images, thanked the woman for her time, and chased the kids down the boardwalk toward Adam's building.

We knocked on Adam's unlocked door and let ourselves in. All four kids barreled through. I heard them squealing, "Grandma! Grandpa! Uncle Adam! Uncle Harrison!" Phil and I followed and greeted his parents with hugs and kisses. Their overly bright smiles seemed unnatural, and I could tell they were nervous as they looked me up and down, searching for signs of distress from my treatment. They had every reason to be concerned for their young, hardworking oldest son. He had a mortgage, four little kids, and a wife undergoing breast cancer treatment, but they fretted over me even more. My mother-in-law had had her own run-in with breast cancer only a few years before and her mother was a two-time breast cancer survivor, so she understood first-hand how stressful it could be.

"Sweetheart," she beamed, her golden charm bracelets jangling as she headed over to give me a hug. She smelled like Perles de Lalique, and her hair was freshly blow-dried. "You look wonderful! And your skin, it's so smooth, great color, too!" Her eyes scanned my fully intact hair and ruddy face, still pink from the wind outside.

"Thanks, Mom, I feel really great," I said, and hoped she could see I meant it.

"You do? Oy, I'm so worried about you, Gila." Her eyes welled up. She caught her tears before they could ruin her mascara. "Here, I bought you something," she sniffled and handed me a flat brown box with an embossed Salvatore Ferragamo logo on the top.

I wasn't one for designer labels, preferring to shop at Zara and Target. But I was touched by her grand gesture, regardless of what was in the box.

"It's something you can use now but also for, um, afterward ..." she trailed off as I removed the lid and saw a large silk scarf printed with colorful illustrations of shoes. It was beautiful. I tied it around my head, pirate style, taking it for a test run. "It looks good on you! But you'll be gorgeous no matter what's on your head," she said while her tears now flowed without hesitation.

"That's nice of you to say, Mom. This is so luxurious, I almost can't wait to have to wear it," I joked and gave her a hug. As tough and fiercely independent as I was, I appreciated being worried about. Sometimes, I just needed to feel like a daughter.

I didn't see the photos from that day until the following week when I sat at the family computer, uploading them from my full SIM card. I zoomed in on the one I thought looked the best until it filled the entire screen. I stared at it for a long time. There we sat in a row, a happy, normal family smiling in the winter sun, the sand and water of Asbury Park beach on the horizon behind us. I was in my uniform of huge sunglasses, denim skirt, sweater, and leather boots, my hair pulled back into a ponytail. None of us knew, not even me, that it was the last photo I'd ever take before my hair started to fall out two days later. I ordered a print and have looked at that photo thousands of times since.

The day my hair started to jump ship was also the date of my second round of chemo, which also happened to be the anniversary of when I got my period for the first time in 1986. I remember it because seventh-grade Gila made a cryptic entry in her homework notebook: "FEB 10 RED" and continued to enter that same uncrackable code on every February 10th page of every homework journal until graduating high school, as if predicting that I'd need to answer the question, "When was your first period?" on a million future medical forms.

Each time I tugged on my hair and nothing came out, I almost allowed myself to believe that I was special, a medical anomaly, but today's yank had finally produced the results I'd been dreading. It wasn't coming out in clumps yet and still looked full because I'd been wearing it curly out of fear of what blow drying it might do, but when I ran my fingers from scalp to tip, they were covered in a network of disembodied strands. My heart rate doubled and a tidal wave of nausea rose in me. I didn't want to spend the next several months shedding all over my house, car, and bed like a Labrador Retriever. I tied my hair back into a low bun hoping that would contain the loose strands for the day and got ready to head into the city.

Effy, one of my two pre-approved chemo chaperones, was on duty to take me to my second round. When he offered to sit with me until I was done, I accepted without hesitation.

"So, I did a little research," he said as we merged onto the New Jersey Turnpike, "and I brought a few things to keep you entertained today." His grin told me he'd brought more than just a few things. His "research," I later found out, included grilling Hayley on what the chemo suite looked like and what might bring me comfort. He also asked Phil about my favorite books and TV shows.

While Effy parked the car, Dr. Seagle took my vitals and put in an order for that hideous red concoction. "You still have your hair!" she noted with surprise, and I beamed. "Most of my patients experience hair loss before their second infusion." Deflated, I confessed that it had started falling out that day and headed out to meet Effy in the waiting room.

Together we walked to my assigned chair and before my rear touched the vinyl seat he said, "Hold on a second!" and, out of his enormous tote bag, pulled a brand-new set of four hundred thread count sheets still in the packaging. I laughed in delight and noticed how much less anxious I felt than the last time. Effy got busy draping the crisp white sheet over the entirety of my chair and stuffing a pillow he'd brought from home into the brand-new pillowcase. A nurse approached—oh crap, it was Rose again!—with several fluid-filled bags and an IV pole and started to set up. Her appearance did not deter Effy from his mission.

"There," he beamed, gesturing for me to sit down, "a throne fit for a germaphobe." He was prone to grand gestures, and I loved it. Grinning, I sank into my luxurious seat. This time, I hardly noticed Rose's mutterings as she hooked me up to the infusion.

When Rose left us to ~~terrorize~~ tend to another patient, Effy continued to unload his bag and I glared at the red river advancing toward my arm. I'd still have preferred to be anywhere else, but at least my terror from two weeks ago was replaced by familiarity and acceptance.

"Here, your favorites." He smiled, fanning out a stack of (also brand-new) *Calvin and Hobbes* and *The Far Side* comic books. "I know because I checked with Phil," he said, clearly pleased with himself. It looked as if he'd bought every single book available in print. I laughed and shook my head in disbelief.

"But wait, there's more," he went on, setting a few cold bottles of an electrolyte drink on my armrest. He then pulled out a portable DVD player, extension cord, and a few DVDs. One of them was *Flight of the Conchords*, a television series starring a New Zealand musical comedy duo who performed under the same name. Their absurdist parody songs made me laugh until I couldn't breathe. Effy set up the DVD and hit play. I made it through a song and a half before my head started to feel slow and foggy. I closed my eyes and for the next few hours, drifted in and out of consciousness.

I don't remember what we talked about and if I did anything undignified, such as fall asleep with my mouth open, but Effy didn't mention it. I do know the day passed exponentially faster with someone there. I slept in the car all the way home and stumbled out onto the sidewalk in front of my house like I was drunk.

I felt boneless, as though someone had stuck a straw in my body and sucked the very life force out of me. Effy walked me to the front door, and I sobbed all the way. "What's this? Gila crying? But you *never* cry!" he joked, invoking my native language: sarcasm. His trick worked and my tears turned into laughter. "This is the best day ever," he went on, "for the rest of your life I'm going to remind you of the one time I saw you cry." It was exactly what I needed at that moment.

Two days later, I went to see Raluca, my longtime hairdresser. "Cut it short. Boy short." Victoria Beckham had recently made waves with a new pixie style, and I allowed myself the fantasy that I'd look just as good.

After drawing a curtain around us for privacy, Raluca tied my hair in a tight ponytail and hacked away just above the elastic hair tie. I planned to shave my head eventually, but while I still had enough hair to work with, a short cut felt like an easier transition into baldness. I wanted to see what I'd look like when my hair started to grow back in.

Tamar and her toddler daughter had come along for moral support and sat on a couch on the other side of the curtain.

"Can I have that, please?" I asked. The disembodied ponytail was placed in my open palm. Raluca gave me a hug and got back to work. Her chrome scissors fluttered around my head while I watched my transformation in the mirror. Staring back at me was Jewish Posh Spice. I would never have opted for a such a close-cropped style, but I had to admit it looked pretty good; it made my brown eyes seem huge and gave my cheekbones more definition. If only it was possible to keep it this way for the duration of my treatment. Raluca refused my attempt to pay her, and I burst into tears. She put her arm around my shoulders and watched me consider my reflection in the mirror.

"I'll be back when I'm ready for you to shave it all off." I sniffled and put on my huge sunglasses, which, in the absence of my usual full head of hair, made me look like a gigantic fly. I stepped past the curtain and into the waiting room, facing Tamar head-on and shaking my head as if to say, "Can you believe this?"

She stood up, towering over me in her black platforms and black puffer coat. Even behind her large (black) sunglasses, I could see she was crying, too.

"It looks good, Gi. I mean it," and I knew she did. I took my camera out of its red leather case and handed it to her.

"Will you take some pictures of me?" I asked, cocking my head to one side and wringing my hands. I had no plans to share the photos with anyone but knew I'd someday want to remember what I looked like that day. We staged a mini photo shoot where I perched on a salon stool and mugged for the camera, even daring to remove my sunglasses for a few shots. Tamar's two-year-old daughter, only a few months older than Kivi, toddled over and looked up at me with her clear, blue eyes. I crouched down to meet her, and Tamar snapped one final photo before I grabbed my brand-new, styled-by-Tova wig out of my bag and positioned it on my head. Using the internal clips, I fastened it to my newly shorn hair and topped it off with my favorite tweed Kangol cap. Tova was wrong and my prediction was right. I did not feel sexy in my wig. I felt whatever the opposite of sexy was. As I left to pick up the kids from school, I wondered how I'd anchor the wig to my head once my hair was all gone.

WHAT NOT TO SAY TO SOMEONE WHO HAS BREAST CANCER THAT PEOPLE ACTUALLY SAID TO ME

How's your white blood cell count? (Shouted from across the street while I was out with my kids.)

I had a mastectomy five years ago and never recovered full range of motion in my arms so don't be surprised if you don't, either. (Don't be surprised when I ghost you.)

I'd give you a hand with the kids, but I just signed up for a silk-screening class on Tuesdays; you have chemo on Tuesdays, right? (Silk. Screening. Class.)

I'd give up the hair on my head if it meant I didn't have to deal with hair removal on the rest of my body. (No, you would not.)

You're so lucky you don't have to waste any time doing your hair, you just throw on your wig and you're out the door! (I hope you're never this "lucky.")

Do you think you got cancer because you ate a lot of soy? (I did not eat a lot of soy.)

It's a good thing you were done having kids anyway. (Eye roll emoji)

Oh, they're so small! I thought they'd be bigger. (You're

welcome to go as big as you like when *you* have a mastectomy and reconstruction.)

Everything happens for a reason! (Literally never *ever* say this
to someone.)

Your mom died, your dad died, and now you have cancer,
too? Surely this means nothing bad will ever happen to
you ever again, you're exempt! (That's not how it works.
Also, don't jinx people.)

Now your hair won't get stuck in your lip gloss. (OK, this
one, from a super campy hairdresser who worked with
Raluca, was funny.)

When *my* _____ had chemo she/he
               (family member/friend/colleague)
had _____ .
    (gross, torturous, undignified side effects)

Hey, it's Tuesday, shouldn't you be in chemo? (Assume that I
have a calendar.)

I thought your skin would be green and bumpy, my mom's
skin was green and bumpy. How is your complexion
still rosy and smooth? (Next time, try "Wow you look
amazing!")

If there's anything I can do to help, let me know. (Don't make
me think of jobs to give you.)

You haven't told your kids? Why not? We don't keep secrets
in *our* family. (Maybe you ought to.)

I could *never* handle everything you're handling, it's too much.
(Yes, you could, you just won't find out until something
bad happens to you.)

It's a good thing your parents aren't here to see this. (True and I agree but STFU.)

Can't you give me more jobs to do? I really want to help. (It's not about you, babe.)

THINGS IT'S OK TO SAY

I'm sorry you're going through this. It really sucks.

Here, I baked this batch of chocolate chip cookies for you.

Would you care to join me on a hike up a mountain, to stand on its peak, and scream into the void until our throats are raw?

I'll be here at 9:00 AM tomorrow to pick up your kids for a full-day outing to the zoo/mall/international space station.

I'm not sure what to say, so I'll take your lead and follow suit accordingly and if that means we talk about everyday mundane things and never once mention your cancer or chemo or wigs or white blood cell count that's A-OK with me.

9

a little death

Lucky for me, fedoras and beanies had always been a part of my signature look because when I picked my kids up from school after getting a pixie cut, they didn't notice anything amiss. Whether I wore it wavy or straight, the "hair" flowing from the brim of my cap was a dead ringer for my own. With my eyebrows and lashes still firmly in place (I checked on those hourly), I still looked exactly like myself. My first few days wearing the wig, even my friends forgot my hair wasn't mine.

The night of haircut day, I waited until the kids were fast asleep before unveiling my new look to Phil. To be on the safe side, I locked our bedroom door and faced him head-on while removing first my hat and then the wig, sending wisps of short hair fluttering to the floor. Most of it was still rooted to my head.

"Beautiful," he said quietly. "Really." This was from a man who I knew was partial to long hair. I let myself believe him, but I still felt ashamed. My best efforts to protect myself from exactly what I was now facing had proven inadequate. I had mammograms and checkups, I exercised regularly and had nursed my kids, I even avoided eating soy products after reading that it might increase the risk of breast cancer (research doesn't support this, by the way!). I had my breasts removed at thirty-four, for crying out loud. I did everything right and still cancer breached my pre-ventative wall. I'd failed to protect myself and, in that, failed to protect Phil from having to worry about my mortality. My short, thinning hair was a stark visual reminder of what was happening, and I hated having him see me that way. It was the last time he'd ever see me without a hat or wig until it grew back. I pulled a soft beanie over my head, kissed Phil goodnight, and went to sleep.

In the morning, I woke up to Ezra and Lea banging on our locked door. Phil went to open it and I held my breath as they ran toward me, terrified they'd be suspicious of the gray knit fabric where my hair usually was. I had my story prepared just in case. "My doctor said I need to take some strong medicine to stay healthy," I'd say, "and sometimes it makes my head very cold!" The only questions they asked were about waffles in the freezer; did we have any and could I warm some up for breakfast. I felt like I'd gotten away with murder.

The following few days were torture. Beneath my wig and hat, my scalp itched like crazy as my hair came loose and got trapped between my scalp and the wig's mesh. I'd take off the head cov-erings at night over the toilet and watch tufts of hair cascade into the bowl. I was amazed that no matter how much came out, I still had what looked like plenty left on my head. My pale scalp was now visible in several places. I looked less like a Spice Girl and more like a rabid racoon that had emerged from a street fight.

"I can't take this anymore, I'm going back to Raluca to have my head shaved tomorrow," I told Phil. It had only been four days since my haircut. I was naïve to think I'd have more time.

"I don't want you to ever see me bald, OK? I don't want that image stuck in your head. I don't even want it stuck in *my* head." I thought of my mother and the things I could never unsee; I desperately wanted to protect my family from that if I could. Lips quivering, I was trying, unsuccessfully, not to cry.

"OK," he said, his eyes getting a bit watery, too. We hugged for a long time, Phil rubbing my back while I wailed into his chest.

My highly realistic plan to preempt my own trauma was this: I'd avoid ever looking in a mirror without something on my head. I was sure if I saw a sick person—or my mother—looking back at me, it would be my undoing. Avoiding my reflection would take a tremendous amount of focus and headspace but would also allow me to dissociate from my new reality. I'd already lost control of so much—this was a small way that I could take hold of what was happening to me. I'd take what I could get.

At Raluca's the next day, I sat with my back to the mirror as she ran her clippers back and forth over my skull.

"You have such a beautiful head shape," she said, a compliment I'd never been given before. I never noticed if my mother's bald head was beautiful. To me, she just looked sick.

"Why thank you," I answered, daring to drag one hand over my skull. It felt like sandpaper, which took me by surprise. I was expecting more "baby's cheek." "Too bad I'll never get to see it," and she laughed, shaking her head.

I slid out of the salon chair and gave her a lopsided smile as we hugged goodbye. There were no tears this time, just resignation and a renewed commitment to my mission to grasp at any shards of normalcy in my upside-down world.

When I tried to position my wig and hat in place again, I was alarmed at how loose they felt. What if a strong wind came and yanked them off? What if I was in a car accident and my head apparatus went through the windshield? Dejected and thoroughly annoyed, I went home to take a nap before school pickup time.

I made it more than three weeks before accidentally catching sight of my hairless head. Mirrors are easy to avoid, shiny chrome shower taps, less so. The inverted sight of myself in the concave base of the tap confused me at first but I quickly realized it was me, all skin tone save for brown eyes and a pink mouth. I nearly slipped and fell from shock. Steadying myself, I wrapped a loose towel around the still-healing scars on my chest and braved a look at myself in the vanity mirror. To my surprise, I felt relief.

My eyebrows and lashes were still fully intact, my skin pink and dewy from the hot shower. I looked like a shop mannequin waiting for someone from the display department to add a hairdo. I did not, as I'd feared, see my mother looking back at me. I saw a powerful woman who was facing her worst fears and saving her life in the process. I laughed in spite of myself, realizing how unnecessarily hard I'd been making things. It would be much easier to work on techniques for securing my hairpieces to a bald head now that I could see what I was doing.

And Raluca was right—I *did* have a nicely shaped head.

My determination to keep my baldness from the kids occupied constant space in my brain whether I noticed it or not, kind of like the hum of a refrigerator. I slept in a close-fitting, soft beret, showered in a puffy plastic cap in case they burst in, as kids are prone to do, and made sure to hide my wig, hat fall, and any related accoutrement high up at the back of my bedroom closet. The best option for securing any hairpiece to a head with no hair for the wig clips to grip was a thin piece of foam sports tape around my head and clamping the clips onto the band.

I'd tried double-sided tape, which did little more than function as wax strips for the tiny black spikes of hair that continued to grow on my scalp even after my head shave. Wandering the sporting goods aisle of Target one day in search of a baseball glove for Ezra, I noticed packages containing brightly colored rolls of foam meant to be tied around elbows and knees to hold sports uniforms in place for safety. With nothing to lose other than $7.99, I bought a roll of pink tape. My investment paid off. Every morning, I'd tear off a twenty-four-inch piece, position the midpoint on top of my head where a headband might rest, and tie it in a tight knot at the base of my skull. I looked like one of those newborn babies in an Anne Geddes photo shoot, but it worked better than anything else I tried and, most importantly, was comfortable.

I could suffer all the side effects privately, without my kids ever detecting anything unusual, except for losing my hair. I threw everything I had into making sure my cover wasn't blown with a careless slipup. I firmly believed—and still do—that there was no value in exposing them to my hair loss, in making them carry that memory forever the way I still did with images of my own mom. Especially since I'd be back to my normal appearance soon and, hopefully, permanently.

For someone who thrived on routine and predictability, I found myself having an awful lot of first-time experiences on my quest to avoid breast cancer. Until a few months earlier, I'd never had surgery, never had an oncologist or chemotherapy, nor the need to wear a wig. Soon I'd have something else to add to that list: For the first time in my nine years of regularly visiting a ritual bath as part of my Jewish faith, I'd be dunking in the mikvah waters without hair.

Married Jewish women visit the mikvah each month after their period stops. A mikvah is sort of like a warm plunge pool in a spa-like facility complete with changing rooms. It's an essential core of religious life and a private matter between spouses. My period arrived the day after my first chemo session and, rather than go for a dunk immediately after it finished, I waited until I shaved my head. The thought of coming up out of the water with my own hairs floating around me like some macabre water dance performance disgusted me. I also knew this would likely be my last visit to a mikvah. During my first meeting with Dr. Seagle to discuss my treatment plan, she'd said that in addition to chemotherapy, I could protect myself from future breast cancer by stopping my estrogen production. First, chemo would halt my period and before it had a chance to return, I'd have my ovaries removed, which would make my menopause permanent.

Although my mother and I never discussed it, I knew she went to the mikvah. The first and only inkling I had of this came when I was seventeen years old. One cold winter night, she came home with soaking wet hair. She avoided making eye contact with me and was hurrying to her bedroom when I intercepted her in the hallway.

Me: Hey Ma, why's your hair wet?

Her: *still no eye contact* I, um, I went swimming.

Me: Really? Where?

If we had access to an indoor pool on Staten Island, I sure didn't know about it.

Her: I don't know. I just went swimming, OK?

And that is a perfect example of the satisfying and emotionally open sorts of conversations I had growing up with my parents.

My first time submerging in a mikvah was the week before my wedding, as is customary for brides. I was excited to take this first step toward married life and when I came up for air to recite the accompanying blessing, I really did feel reborn. A better version of myself. A version that was about to marry a great guy and live in holy matrimony on the Upper West Side.

As life got busier with kids, going to the mikvah (and the meticulous cleaning of the body in preparation) became less exciting and more of an inconvenience. Once a month may not sound like a lot but with an ever-growing to-do list, it felt like mikvah night was coming around every five minutes. I was fully committed to upholding the age-old ritual but sometimes (often) fantasized about the onset of menopause.

How many times had I wished to be freed of this obligation? And now here I was, a cautionary tale about being careful what you wish for, going to the mikvah one last time, already nostalgic for what I'd soon lose.

Like my first visit as a bride, this one seemed to function as a separation between life stages: between my fertile, feminine years and my ailing self who, despite her best efforts, hadn't managed to dodge cancer. I checked with my oncologist first to make sure that I wasn't exposing my immunocompromised body to anything dangerous by going into the water naked. I'd never before needed medical permission to go to the mikvah; having to ask forced me to acknowledge my citizenship in the land of illness.

A specially trained female mikvah attendant escorted me from my assigned waiting room where I completed my preparation (removal of jewelry, nail polish, contact lenses, or anything else not belonging to my body) to a small room, the main feature of which was a tiny plunge pool with a set of stairs. My incisions—hip to hip, under the arm, and from the nipple to below each breast were still red and raw and angry. Until recently, they'd been weeping but had finally stopped. Even though the mikvah was kept highly chlorinated, I had to be extra careful about infection.

The attendant turned away while I removed my white terry robe and wool beanie. On past visits, the attendant would turn back around only to check that I was fully underwater, as was required. This time I asked her to make an exception.

"Would you mind keeping your back to me while I go under?" I said as I made my way down the stairs until my feet touched the floor. The warm water rippled as I walked to the center. "I'll be able to feel when I'm completely submerged." I was embarrassed by my baldness and although she made no mention of it, I knew she understood the reason for my request.

"Of course," her voice echoed off the tiled walls, "take your time and let me know when you're out."

Instead of it feeling like a rebirth, a purification by water, it felt like a little death. My fresh surgical scars and exposed scalp changed the experience entirely. I stayed below the surface a beat longer than usual and opened my mouth wide as if to let out a silent scream. Were it not for the attendant I'd have screamed for real, creating a jacuzzi with my bubbles of rage. I came up for air, my eyes stinging from the tears I'd held behind squeezed lids and recited the Al Hatvilah blessing, which sanctified the act of submerging. It was the only time I ever cried underwater.

10

getting all chemotional

Life quickly fell into a rhythm around chemotherapy. It's amazing what you can get used to when you have no choice. My all-day infusions took place every other Tuesday, but Tamar and another friend who was also named Gila, took my two older kids for sleepovers every Tuesday. Neither Ezra, who was seven, nor Lea, five, ever questioned why the universe saw fit to grant them sleepovers on a school night *every single week for four months*. I, however, thanked God every day for giving me children smart enough to not look a gift horse in the mouth.

Aside from my shot of Neulasta, administered by Tamar, I spent every other Wednesday in bed. Don't be jealous; I didn't choose the chemo life, the chemo life chose me.

Most days, I drove the kids to school even though it was only around the corner from our house. My cavernous Nissan Quest served as a barrier between me and unwelcome questions about my health from people who forgot, no matter how many times I reminded them, that my kids didn't know I was in treatment. I made suppers of chicken fingers and rice, turkey burgers, or mac and cheese whenever I felt up to it. At night, with the exception of treatment days when I felt like a husk of a human, I'd bathe the kids and read to them at bedtime, often falling asleep next to Tani, whose trundle bed pulled out from under Ezra's. Nothing made me feel more normal, more at peace, than our nightly ritual. When the boys fell asleep, I'd bury my face in their necks and luxuriate in the mingled scents of Downy fabric softener and Colgate Berry Blast toothpaste from their puffs of breath before going to do the same with Lea and Kivi in their bedrooms.

Tamar stopped by every day and brought regards from people in the community who asked to visit. She'd check with me before allowing anyone in, like my own personal bouncer. Miryam and Mikey often came for Shabbat or took the kids to their Upper West Side apartment, and Rivky and I spoke on the phone often. She lived in Queens, was pregnant with her second child, and had a one-year-old to look after, so I turned down her many offers to drive in to help me. As tempted as I was to let her come clean my house before Passover, I was still the big sister and couldn't accept. My little sister had enough on her plate.

Somewhere between my third and fourth doses of Adriamycin-Cytoxan I started to have symptoms of neuropathy, which caused numbness in my hands and feet. Thanks to my gigantic yellow Emend pills, I never became nauseous. And not to brag, but I never even got one mouth sore! What I did get was an icy, frozen sensation from my nose down to my chin meaning when I spoke it felt like I'd just come in from a two-hour walk in a snowstorm. It's what I imagined Botox must feel like.

Phil and I celebrated my halfway point after my fourth round of chemo by going out for pizza and a movie. I don't remember what we saw, but I do remember how I felt as I lay my head on Phil's shoulder: tired, protected, and sick to death of wearing my stupid wig. It felt like a thousand ants were performing Riverdance under my hat.

Round five marked the end of my fruit punch chemo regimen and the first dose of Taxol, which was supposedly gentler than Adriamycin-Cytoxan and didn't cause hair loss, not that I had any left to lose anywhere on my body. And when I say anywhere, I very much mean *anywhere*. The few strays that seemed to cling on for dear life I regarded with curiosity and reverence. From a Darwinian point of view, I had to admire these hangers-on, clearly made of tougher stuff than their fallen brethren.

Taxol had a high incidence of causing allergic reactions, so before I could start my drip, I had to have a steroid administered by IV as a precaution. The steroid was called Decadron, which sounded like a Transformer, making me laugh until about ten minutes in when I became so violently nauseous I started retching and doubling over on my sheet-covered chair. It was ten times worse than the morning sickness I had with each of my pregnancies, and I was so out of control, I peed myself a little. The indignity of it all made me start crying through the gagging and the peeing and I was just grateful that it was Hayley, not Effy, on duty that day. I felt sorry for Hayley having to bear witness to my misery.

At the first signs of hair loss, I started obsessively inspecting my eyebrows and lashes, taking note of how sparse they were getting. I'd tug at them like a masochist and was heartbroken at how easily they came loose from my face. One morning, after the kids had gone to school but before Phil had left for the office, I stood in the downstairs bathroom and stared at myself in the mirror. Instead of my usual beret or gray fedora, I wore the Ferragamo silk scarf tied across my forehead to anchor the wig in place. The scarf looked cool but lacked the coverage a hat brim provided, and my face felt exposed in a way I didn't like.

"I have no eyebrows left, no lashes. If my skin turns green, I'll literally look like a cartoon alien," I fumed. I was exaggerating, of course. They'd thinned a lot but, to anyone's eye other than my own, plenty still remained. Phil walked up behind me and considered my reflection.

"If you had as much hair on your upper lip as you have above your eyes, you'd be running to get it waxed off," he mused.

"Fair point," I admitted, and turned to kiss him before stomping upstairs to apply some brown eyeshadow to my brows. Damn Phil for always knowing the right thing to say.

Sometimes while reading, a few lash and brow hairs would flutter down into my book. You'd think they wouldn't make a sound as they hit the page, but you'd be wrong. To me, they sounded like a jackhammer, like glass shattering, a sonic boom. For a while, I collected the tiny strands of dislodged hair in a Ziploc bag like a beauty salon serial killer storing trophies. Was I planning to glue them back onto my face? I don't know. I just knew I wasn't ready to let them go.

Hayley and Effy's campaign to outdo each other in their chaperone duties waged on, which delighted me to no end.

Hayley brought stacks of magazines, flowers, and sheets with an even higher thread count than Effy's. She also had a word with the head nurse and finally had Rose replaced with someone with better interpersonal skills. Effy accepted my challenge to bring me a falafel from my favorite place on Ben Yehuda Street in Jerusalem and, on my sixth chemo, handed me a small box that had an Israeli return address and postage markings. He was practically giddy as he watched me open the box and take out what looked and smelled very much like a delicious falafel. Did he not realize I was immunocompromised and that eating a three-day-old sandwich that had traveled six thousand miles in the underbelly of an airplane could kill me?

"I'm not eating this," I said, even though the falafel looked suspiciously intact. "You're nuts."

"You asked for a Jerusalem falafel, and I delivered! Next time give me a harder challenge!"

He finally told me the falafel was fresh; he'd ordered it to the hospital from a kosher restaurant in New York while I was slumped over during my infusion that morning and tucked it into a box he'd had his brother in Jerusalem ship to him, empty, for this purpose. I dug in, savoring not only the delicious snack but also my good fortune in having a friend who'd go to such lengths just to get a smile out of me.

During chemotherapy, I continued to see Elisheva for weekly massages at her studio near my house. It had dim lights, plants in crocheted macramé holders hanging from hooks in the ceiling, and burgundy walls stacked with shelves covered in protective talismans. A pink and orange batik print scarf that stretched across the ceiling was both trippy and soothing, and the room smelled of patchouli and roasted sunflower seeds.

At first, I was self-conscious of Elisheva seeing my bald head, so I wore a beanie while she massaged me from the neck down. Finally, one day around the halfway mark of my chemotherapy, I climbed onto her table, lay my head down, and peeled off my hat.

"Here," I said, passing it to her. Elisheva took my hat and held both hands to her heart.

"*Merveilleux*!" she sang, "You 'old so much tension in your 'ead, now I can really 'elp you!"

"I know you can," I said, closing my eyes as she positioned herself behind me and started kneading my skull. It was so good, I felt like an idiot for robbing myself of the pleasure until now.

"Your 'ead eez a very beautiful shape, you know?" she mused.

"You're not the first person to tell me that," I laughed, before drifting off into a state of half sleep.

With Elisheva, I allowed myself to be vulnerable. I'd whimper and sometimes full-on bawl before and after our sessions, knowing that my anguish wouldn't be a burden to her because she'd do some spiritual trick, like visualize it as a leaf and send it down the river or whatever, and we'd both be free of my heaviness.

In mid-March, I got a cold. Which I ignored. Because that's what I'd always done. Why would I make a big deal about a cold? What was I, a man? I needed to believe I was still strong enough to enjoy the luxury of having a garden-variety, seasonal cold without any further consequences. To worry about a cold would be to acknowledge that I was, in fact, immunocompromised. The holiday of Purim was only a couple days away and I'd be damned if I was going to let anyone or anything keep me from celebrating the most joyous of Jewish holidays, the one where it's customary to dress up in costumes. Esther, the heroine of the Purim story, hides her identity so we hide ours, too. Finally, a day when I wouldn't be the only one who didn't look like myself.

I'd got to thinking about hidden miracles like the ones in the Purim story—hidden identities and reversals of fortune—through a new lens. Being Jewish meant believing in some things I could not see, and this extended to my belief that the hand of God was working invisibly in the background and that wherever I was at any moment was exactly where I was meant to be. Phil had posed the idea of a move to London many times before, but I'd never agreed until recently. That decision had set my theoretical plan for a double mastectomy in motion and not a moment too soon. That was not happenstance. I thought about my recent close call, how my tiny, aggressive tumors, although contained within my breast, were positioned one millimeter away from my chest wall. Had I waited any longer to have the mastectomy, they'd have infiltrated the rest of my body. My prognosis would have been poor, and my problems would be considerably more severe than a cold ruining my Purim.

The kids and I baked traditional Purim hamantaschen, triangle cookies filled with prune butter that no one liked except for me and Phil. I used my mother's recipe. Holding the recipe card written in her loopy cursive made me feel a little more connected to her. I rarely spoke to my kids about my mom, but once a year we baked Babi Faigie's hamantaschen. That's what I wanted my kids to call her even though they'd never met this grandmother: Babi a classic Eastern European term for Grandma.

Purim was on a Tuesday this year, but luckily, not a chemo Tuesday. Our friends hosted a huge Purim feast for twenty families in a big white tent in their driveway and the kids and I went dressed as Lego people in costumes I'd made by hand. I made each of them a large Lego helmet out of Styrofoam and colorful felt. For myself, I made a 2D hairpiece out of yellow cardboard and positioned it to frame my face and obscure the edges of my wig. I hid my wig with a wig. It was pure genius.

There was still a bite to the March air, and I bundled up in a warm coat and gloves. Still, by the time we returned home that night, I felt pretty run-down and knew I'd stood out in the cold too long. I wasn't prone to contracting colds or viruses, though a small thought kept bubbling up: *You're halfway into an atomic chemo regimen, maybe your resistance isn't quite at its normal level.* But I put that thought in a slingshot, drew it way back, and let go, sending it rocketing into the next stratosphere.

The next day, Phil took the kids to school and made me promise to take it easy.

"Stay in bed today, OK? No trips to Target or buying stuff for London. OK?" It was March and our move was still five months away, but every minute I focused on preparations for my future was a minute I didn't have to think about my present.

I promised. On his way out, Phil reminded me of his plans to meet some old friends in the city for drinks after work.

"Call me if you need me to come home, I'll jump in a car service." He looked worried.

"I'll be fine, hon, you go ahead and enjoy. You need a break," I assured him even as I felt a cold sheen of sweat collect on my forehead.

Phil was capable of shouldering more than his fair share. But even someone with the ability to balance all-nighters at the office, communal obligations like leading prayer services on Shabbat, and family plans like Sunday outings needed a break. As the husband, Phil was expected to serve as head of PR on my cancer task force and answer the questions, "How's she doing?" and "How are the kids coping?" wherever he went. Most didn't think to ask him how *he* was doing. He needed a support system, too, which had nothing to do with me. I was happy for him to get together with friends and blow off some steam. His suffering may not have been the same as mine, but I knew that his burden was just as great.

By the time the kids went to bed, I could no longer ignore how crappy I felt: shivering, sweating, aching bones, just like the cancer characters in movies and TV shows. They were always huddled under a blanket, bald and gray-faced with chattering teeth. Since day one, I took great pains to never look like those people, and instead to be the poster child for how great someone undergoing chemo could look. Chemo patients: they're just like us!

Every morning, I took time and care to draw on my eyebrows, to fill in my sparse lash line with dark powder, and to swipe a few coats of thickening mascara on what lashes remained. Like the wig, makeup had not been a part of my daily routine prior to chemo. Now I relied on it to protect my kids from my reality.

At that particular moment, however, I was feeling decidedly unchic. I popped a few Advil, chugged a glass of water, then sat at the kitchen table willing myself to feel better. Dr. Seagle's face materialized before me like a hologram. Her soft, synthesized voice delivered the same directive she'd leave me with at the end of our biweekly pre-chemo check-ins: "If you get a fever, call my office immediately."

Fever in a chemo patient could be a sign of infection, and infection in a body with a weakened immune system could quickly spread and lead to sepsis.

As a seasoned mom, I could detect whether my kids had fever by kissing their foreheads. I couldn't kiss my own forehead and for a fleeting moment, I wished my mom was there to do it for me, but I instinctively knew, the way I know when my kids are lying about having brushed their teeth, that I was burning up with fever. I probably just needed some antibiotics, I told myself. Instead of calling my doctor, I called Phil.

"Hey, who do we know who can get me some antibiotics this late at night?" I asked through chattering teeth.

Without missing a beat, Phil said, "I'm calling Benjy to take you to his hospital. I'll meet you there."

"Don't c-c-come to the hospital, I'll p-p-probably be home before you anyway." My shivering had reached the same intensity as the final spin cycle on an old washing machine.

"Gila. Could you just for once in your life not be so stubborn? Jeez. I'm meeting you there. I'll call you back to confirm that Benjy's coming."

"I'm sorry I ruined your n-n-night."

"You know for someone so smart, you can be pretty dumb sometimes."

"I love you."

"I love you, too," and he hung up.

I remembered what Benjy had said while he removed my final surgical drain way back in December: "I'm the head of an emergency room, that might come in handy. Don't hesitate to call if you need help." He reminded Phil of this whenever their paths crossed in shul on Shabbat. Benjy called me less than a minute after Phil hung up.

"Looks like we're going on a little adventure! I'll be over in three minutes. Do you have someone to watch the kids?"

I called Tamar, who was on her way before I hung up the phone.

My wig was upstairs in my bedroom, and I didn't have the energy to get it, so I'd be going out in public sans hairpiece for the first time. I was such a mess, I didn't even care. Besides, Benjy being an ER doctor had certainly seen people who looked worse than me. I grabbed a black Yankees baseball cap from a hook at the front door and jammed it on top of the bandana already on my head. Convincing myself that this gave me a sort of gangster quality rather than just a thirty-five-year-old mom going to the hospital in middle of the night, I pushed my aching arms into the sleeves of my puffer coat while squinting through the front door peephole. Benjy was already standing on the porch. When I opened the door, he was grinning like Lady Luck herself had dragged him out of his nice warm house on a freezing night in early spring. Just then, Tamar came running up my driveway, resplendent in her black sweatpants and hoodie.

"I'm so sorry I had to get you out at this hour—" I started to say to Tamar, but she rolled her eyes and brushed past me on her way to the kitchen.

"Just go take care of yourself, I'll be right here reorganizing your freezer and spice cabinet," she said, shooing me off.

I stepped outside, now shivering even harder.

"Is that your car?" I asked through clenched teeth, nodding at the black Corvette parked in front of my house. I'd only ever seen Benjy riding around town with his family in a minivan like the rest of us.

"This is my fun car. I felt the occasion called for it," he said, opening the passenger door. I'd never been in a Corvette before. It would have been cool if I wasn't on my way to the emergency room with a possibly life-threatening infection.

"Are you sure I can't just get some antibiotics and stay home?" I tried. "I don't want you to spend your night in the hospital for nothing," but he wouldn't hear of it.

Benjy kept the conversation light and airy, even getting me to laugh a few times during the ten-minute ride and I started to wonder if he was doing that thing doctors do when they know you're in hot water, but don't want to make you panic so they employ distraction tactics. If that was the case, it was working.

He'd called ahead, and the way the staff fawned over me when we arrived, I understood how highly regarded Benjy was in this hospital. I was whisked into an examination room, had my blood drawn, and was offered a cup of tea while I waited for the results. They came back faster than I thought possible. A girl could really get used to this kind of VIP treatment.

A young woman in green scrubs burst into the exam room, her eyes wide and mouth agape in horror. She was holding a printout of my lab report, and blurted, "Your white blood cell count, it's off the charts!"

Her alarm turned to confusion when Benjy and I barely reacted. We exchanged a knowing look before he turned to her saying, "It's OK, Irene, Mrs. Pfeffer is a chemo patient, so the elevated white blood cells are from the Neulasta in her system." Grabbing a pen from his shirt pocket, he scribbled something on an oversize pad, asked me if I was allergic to penicillin, and when I said no, continued scribbling before tearing off the sheet and handing it to Irene whose color was slowly returning to her face.

"Let's get Mrs. Pfeffer on a high-dose Amoxicillin drip and then send her home with a seven-day course to be taken orally."

"I *told* you I just needed some antibiotics," I muttered under my breath. Benjy heard and laughed.

"Maybe you should consider a career in medicine," he joked.

Fifteen minutes later, I sat resting my head against the wall as the amoxicillin dripped into my arm. I reached for my phone to give Phil an update when the door opened and he poked his head in. The poor guy was out of breath and even though his glasses were fogged over from running in from the cold, I could see how worried he was. Phil looked worse than Irene had when she thought I was going into sepsis. He might have even looked worse than me.

"I told you I'd meet you at the hospital," he said, kissing me lightly with freezing lips.

"I told you not to," and he chuckled. I draped my free arm, the one without an IV line in it, around his neck.

"Did you have fun tonight? Until I wrecked it, I mean."

"Yes. I had fun."

"More fun than this?" I deadpanned, and he laughed.

He pulled up a chair and we sat side by side in silence, our heads resting on one another until the antibiotic bag was empty and Benjy swooped into the room and said, "You two kids about ready to head home?"

The fever was the one major setback in my otherwise run-of-the-mill four months of chemo and while I'd have preferred to have had zero complications (or better yet, zero need for chemotherapy), I knew how lucky I was compared to women undergoing the same treatment and whose lives hung in the balance. I finally understood what Dr. Seagle had meant when she referred to my need for chemo as a huge inconvenience. To other patients, she may have presented it as a matter of life and death. And it wasn't just my stellar prognosis that put me at an advantage. I had Phil and did not take for granted how much easier my ordeal was with him by my side. I wondered how my mother might have fared if she'd had a Phil of her own.

One night in mid-April, before my second-to-last infusion, I pulled out my mother's medical file and lay in bed flipping through the pages. In the decade and a half since her death, I'd read it a hundred times, but always through the eyes of someone who'd never had a cancer. Now as I skimmed, I landed on the words "Adriamycin," "Cytoxan," and "Taxol." I was having the exact same treatment (ACT) as my mom had seventeen years earlier. I'd taken every precaution possible to avoid cancer and she'd taken zero, yet here I was in the same boat as her. I was livid.

"It says here that my mom had the exact same chemo cocktail I'm having now!" I scoffed. Phil was next to me, trying to watch TV. With his attention still on the screen, he gave me a sideways glance.

"I mean, that's what they use to treat breast cancer, which applies in both your cases, so . . ." he answered, treading carefully. "But hers was advanced, Stage III! She didn't even go for mammograms. I've been on top of my health from day one. I did everything right! What do I get for that?" I was nearly hysterical now. Phil turned to face me head-on. He cocked his head to one side and without missing a beat, said, "You get to live."

I'd become comfortable enough in my chemo routine to make a few exceptions to the "Hayley and Effy only" rule. On an Effy day, Miryam left her midtown office to spend her lunch break with me. She brought steak and mashed potatoes in takeout containers from one of my favorite restaurants. Effy excused himself to make a phone call and to give us some time alone. My diagnosis had prompted Miryam to go for gene testing and she'd recently gotten the results of her BRCA test. She was a carrier. Immediately afterward, she decided to have a preventative mastectomy, too. My cancer had thrown her for a loop, and she worried about starting a family with the threat of breast cancer looming over her, the one that had followed me ever since my mother's death. My diagnosis passed that threat on to Miryam.

"I met with Dr. Giannaros and Dr. Maitlin this week," she confided. "We talked about doing silicone implants for reconstruction." At five foot two inches and what I would guess around one hundred pounds, my petite sister had the flat stomach of a twenty-nine-year-old whose body hadn't yet been through the ringer of pregnancy. She had no fat for a TRAM Flap.

"I'm telling you, Gi, I was losing sleep deciding whether to have the surgery now or wait. The minute I decided to go for it, I felt so much better. I'd rather have kids a little bit later and know I'll be there for them," she mused. "You were my wake-up call."

I welled up with pride and vindication. Miryam had initially supported my decision to have a preventative mastectomy but insisted she'd never have one herself. In saving my own life, I might well have been saving hers, too. Maybe Rivky and Gita would follow our lead. It felt like I was finally keeping the promise I made to our mother on her death bed.

"Well, you're welcome," I smiled, picking at my mashed potatoes and wishing I was hungrier. "That's what big sisters are for."

She had her double mastectomy in the same hospital I did a

few weeks before I completed my chemo. Believe it or not, her recovery room was the only empty one on a floor filled with the entourage of another Middle Eastern prince. My only regret was that I was in no physical or immunological shape to offer her any support while she recovered. When her pathology came back clear, I wept with relief.

The day before my eighth and final chemo session, I had a brilliant idea: I would skip it altogether. I wanted to differentiate myself from my mother in some small way (aside from not dying, of course); I wanted a reward for having been so dutifully vigilant about my health for so long. I remembered Dr. Seagle's words during our first meeting: "You could walk out of here and never come back and probably be fine." Although my mother and I had the same chemo to treat the same type of breast cancer, hers was administered as a neoadjuvant—a first step to shrink a tumor before the main treatment, which was surgery. Mine was prescribed as a precaution. There was nothing to shrink. By the time the first drop of Crystal Light Fruit Punch had entered my vein, my tumors had long since left the building. Still, I was so angry that despite my best efforts, I'd had to endure the very thing the preventative mastectomy was meant to save me from, and I wanted to distinguish my experience from hers in some way. We were not the same.

I called Dr. Seagle the day before and requested permission to skip the eighth round.

She was unequivocal in her answer: yes. "Missing this last one, given your case, won't make any difference. Even if down the road you have a reoccurrence, it will have nothing to do with whether or not you missed your last one." Finally, an answer I was happy with.

Phil, however, was not happy when I made my case that night over dinner.

"There's a reason the regimen was set at eight rounds and not seven, Gi. I know you're sick of this and I want you to be past it, too, and it's your decision, but . . ." He had a pained look on his face while he pushed his food around his plate.

"I *really* don't want it," I said, getting up for a second helping of lasagna.

"I know."

"I don't want to sit in that chair or be in that room or have to walk past a row of sick, bony women anymore. I've put in my time; I'm done with that place." I stood over the Pyrex dish on the stovetop, took a huge forkful and shoveled it into my mouth. Another side effect I hadn't experienced throughout my treatment was loss of appetite.

"I know," he said again.

"I'll go into the city tomorrow and decide once I'm there."

"OK." He pulled me in for a hug and let out a long, shaky sigh. I knew then I'd have that last infusion because if I didn't, Phil would worry about me for the rest of his days. I'd do it for him. It's not like I was going to get any balder.

On a warm day in early May, I entered the chemo suite for the last time and was surprised at how triumphant I felt. I was a different person than when I'd first entered in January and while I wasn't about to sit down and have a few beers with the oncology staff to reminisce about the good (bad) times, I allowed myself a sense of accomplishment. I'd endured the thing that scared me most, the thing I thought would be, for me, unendurable.

Hayley, who came with me to the first round, was also with me for the last one. Late that afternoon, a nurse unhooked me from the final empty bag of Taxol, and removed the cannula from my vein. I was free to leave and never come back. If it wouldn't have been insensitive to the women waiting for news or treatment, I'd have broken out into spontaneous song. Hayley would have joined me, too. She has an excellent singing voice and isn't embarrassed to act like an ass in public. It's one of her best qualities. On our way to the elevator, I heard my name being called. It was Dr. Seagle standing in the doorway between the waiting area and the examining rooms, just as she had the first time I met her. She still looked like a fifteen-year-old wearing a white lab coat, albeit a coat being pushed to the limit by the very pregnant belly beneath. I was relieved that she hadn't gone into labor before my final round.

"I just came out to say goodbye and congrats!" she said. I told Hayley I'd meet her in the lobby and walked across the waiting area to Dr. Seagle. (Bye-bye, coffee machine! So long, overstuffed striped sofas pretending to be a living room rather than a cancer club! Hasta la vista, stacks of pamphlets on how to alleviate neuropathy and mouth sores! It was like *Goodnight Moon: Cancer Edition*.) She invited me into her office.

"It's been a pleasure getting to know you," she said. "I want to wish you lots of luck with your oophorectomy and your move to London. Let me know if you need any letters or reports to take with you. And please do keep in touch!"

I promised I would.

I thanked her for her care and for treating me with respect and dignity. Sometimes I forgot I was her patient rather than her friend. I wished her good luck for the birth, and we hugged goodbye around her belly.

I may have been finished with chemotherapy, but I was only one-third of the way into a three-pronged offensive against a recurrence. The next two phases were surgically removing my ovaries and fallopian tubes (bilateral salpingo-oophorectomy, if you must know) followed by a prescription for an aromatase inhibitor, a daily pill that blocks the remaining traces of estrogen produced by a small gland even once the ovaries have been removed. Being a BRCA1 carrier meant I was at high risk for ovarian cancer. When my results came in and I decided to have the preventative mastectomy, I also decided to have my ovaries removed, but assumed I could wait until I was forty. Since breast cancer had been present in my body, it was critical that I stop all estrogen production in my body to prevent a recurrence. I was thirty-five and didn't mind moving the procedure up by a few years. I'd had my kids and, however bad the symptoms of menopause might be, I figured they couldn't be any worse than how I'd felt during chemo.

11

technically a woman

My body needed a medical break between finishing chemo and going back into the hospital for my oophorectomy, but by no means did I rest. We were about to move to London.

Six days after I strode out of the breast oncology center for the last time, Phil and I flew to London for a four-day pilot trip. We met with a realtor who showed us so many rental houses, it made me dizzy. Or maybe that was because I'd taken a transatlantic overnight flight and was running around trying to set up a life in London eight days after having a final round of toxic chemicals forced into my bloodstream. I guess we'll never know! We chose a small, semi-detached house around the corner from the school our kids would attend and headed back to New Jersey.

Once back, I had a consult with Dr. Bradford, a gynecological oncologist (try saying that three times fast) who Dr. Seagle had referred. He'd be carrying out phase two of my three-phase plan to keep breast cancer at bay for good, which was the removal of my ovaries. The TRAM Flap procedure left me nipple-less and Dr. Bradford asked whether I might like Dr. Maitlin to attend my oophorectomy and fashion some nipples while I was already under general anesthesia. I hadn't been bothered enough by the Barbie-like appearance of my post-surgical breasts to undergo yet more surgery just to have some nips slapped on, but now I was being offered a two-for-one and thought, sure, why not?

I sat across from Dr. Bradford as he scanned my medical chart. I knew he'd gotten to the good part when he stopped, looked up with wide eyes and delivered the line I'd come to expect by then: "You know you saved your own life, right?" I sure do, buddy.

He explained the outpatient procedure in which he would use a laparoscope to locate and suck out my ovaries through small slits in the scar tissue on my hips. Dr. Maitlin would use some tissue from the same area to make the functionless but aesthetically pleasing nipples. It was very efficient.

We set a date in June, shook hands, and I went out into the waiting room with yet another clipboard filled with forms to complete and sign. On one of the documents, I came across a checkbox authorizing the surgeon to also remove my uterus, cervix, and some other neighboring organs if necessary. I knocked on Dr. Bradford's office door to ask what was up with the fire sale on my organs.

"Oh, that's in case we find any cancer when we go in," he said casually, as if he wasn't voicing aloud my deepest nightmare scenario. He wasn't insensitive, he was simply being direct and couldn't have known how tightly wound I was, how much latent trauma I carried from that Thanksgiving phone call.

"Why would you need to take any other organs out even in the event you found cancer?"

"Staging!" he said brightly, as if it was obvious. I pictured myself lying on the OR table, a red velvet theater curtain behind me and a spotlight trained on my open torso. A ragtime musical number begins to play and one by one, my ovaries, uterus, liver, and pancreas climb out. They hold silver-tipped canes and wear tiny top hats as they kick their way across my body, singing the final bars of "Hello My Baby" before dropping to their knees and doing jazz hands to the applause of Dr. Bradford and his team.

"What do you mean by 'staging'?" I asked, genuinely confused. He explained that if my ovaries turned out to show signs of cancer, the rest of my reproductive parts would have to be removed in order to determine what stage my cancer was in. I was sorry I asked.

In mid-June, Kivi turned two and we threw a birthday party at our house. When you're two and haven't yet started school, your friendship circle is pretty small. There were plenty of kids at the party, though, cousins or our friends' kids, including Tamar's daughter, the one who'd seen me right after my short haircut. In photos from that day, I look downright joyful. I'm holding Kivi on my mostly healed hip while everyone sings Happy Birthday, posing with Tamar and our kids in the kitchen, and then with Phil's grandma Sylvia, known as GG to our kids, laughing while trying to wrestle myself away from Phil who has his arms playfully around my waist. And I was happy at this first family gathering since I'd survived hell.

My imminent bilateral salpingo-oophorectomy didn't terrify me as much as my other two surgeries had—perhaps because it was my third time going under general anesthesia in eight months. More than anything though, I felt a sense of impending loss that hadn't hit me when I had my breasts removed. Although the mastectomy was a much longer, more involved operation, it was essentially a cosmetic procedure. It didn't lead to any physiological changes in my body. Having my ovaries removed would make permanent the menopause that chemo had started. I'd already experienced plenty of symptoms while undergoing treatment, it was hard to differentiate between what was the medicine's side effects and what was a lack of hormones.

Above all, the choice to have a mastectomy was empowering. It was a trailblazing move at the time and one that ultimately forced friends and family to take their own breast health more seriously. The removal of my ovaries felt less like a choice. Sure, I could have refused to have them out until I was forty, as I'd originally planned when I tested positive for BRCA1, but that would not have been in keeping with my attitude toward prevention. My mother's refusal to heed her doctor's directive to have a mastectomy filled me with what-ifs and still does today.

What bothered me the most, however, was the possibility that Dr. Bradford, Dr. Maitlin, and their teams would see me bald. I was done with chemo, but with no hair, I still presented as a chemo patient and there was nothing I could do about it. The thought of my surgical cap moving during surgery and my scalp being exposed was an indignity I couldn't bear. I tried to wear my wig and scarf into the OR, but no dice. In the end, we compromised, and I wore my scarf tied tightly on my head and *on top* of that, the stupid puffy hair cap. When I woke up in a recovery cubicle next to Phil, the first thing I noticed was how sore my chest felt. I'd almost forgotten that I was getting new nipples that day, too. First though, I patted the front and sides of my head and realized my scarf was askew.

Phil looked drained and I had to remind myself that while I was the one having to repeatedly go under the knife, at least I got to sleep through the ordeal. This was the third time he'd spent his day pacing the hospital halls, waiting for the news from a surgeon that his wife was OK. But I had more pressing matters to address.

"When they wheeled me out here was my head covered?" I demanded.

"Yes, hon." He exhaled, rubbing his temples and shaking his head at his control freak of a wife.

"You didn't see me bald?"

"No, hon," he said convincingly enough that despite my suspicions that my head wrap had been removed and replaced while I'd been unconscious, I let it go.

"And by the way," he went on in a tone of controlled calm, "in case you're interested, I spoke to Dr. Bradford before you woke up and he said everything looked clear. He doesn't expect the pathology to show anything, either."

"Oh. Well, that's good. Can we go home now? I'm starving."

There's a scene in the film *Erin Brockovich* where Erin visits a woman called Donna, who has been harmed by the carcinogenic chemicals an energy company has dumped into the local water supply. Donna has had multiple surgeries for the resulting cancer. She's a young mother in her thirties and is trying to grapple with the betrayal by the corporation and the devastating impact it's had on her body.

Donna asks Erin, "You think that if you got no uterus and no breasts, you're still technically a woman?" and Erin, her voice soft with compassion and sisterhood, answers, "Sure you are. Yeah, you just . . . you're actually a happier woman because you don't have to worry about maxi-pads and underwire."

After my oophorectomy, when I wasn't doubled over in pain from post-surgical gas, I thought about this scene a lot. I had no breast tissue, no hair, no fertility, and most of my torso was covered in scars and sutures, but I didn't feel any less like a woman.

Phil never missed a chance to tell me I was beautiful. From the way he looked at me, I knew he meant it. I was a mother who stopped at nothing to make sure she could continue her role. There was a lot of power in that.

I bled for several days and when it was over, I had the overwhelming urge to go to the mikvah. I knew it wasn't menstrual blood, that it was post-surgical fluids, and that I was not required to go, but it felt like the last chance I would have. Going to the mikvah this time would be purely for me. It was a chance to bring closure to the part of my life that had given me children, femininity, a chance to participate in an ancient ritual just like the generations of women before me. But in the absence of an obligation to go, I consulted our rabbi to see if it was permissible. "Absolutely, you can go. Do everything as you normally would, just don't say the blessing," he said, referring to the words I'd typically recite to sanctify the ritual. My submersion would be purely symbolic, but this wasn't an empty or wasted ritual. It was a chance to feel normal again. I went, still hairless and cramping a bit from surgery and dunked once then twice more, without a blessing. This time, rather than a rebirth, I emerged feeling like my slate had been wiped clean, as though I'd marked the end of my cancer treatment with a watertight seal.

Our August 17 moving date was fast approaching. Our furniture and worldly possessions had already been packed into a forty-foot container that was now somewhere in the Atlantic Ocean on its way to England. A few weeks before we left, Adam threw us a bon voyage party at his Asbury Park apartment. Gita had recently returned from her gap year in Jerusalem; it was the first time all four of my siblings and I had been together in forever, and it was quite the sight to see my kids with all their cousins. They numbered eleven altogether; our family was rebuilding itself one kid at a time. Our family and friends came out to celebrate and send us off the best way they knew how: with a lavish spread of bagels, lox, cheese boards, and a fruit platter, all expertly prepared by Adam and my mother-in-law. The adults clinked L'chaim with glasses of perfectly chilled Sancerre and highballs of Bloody Marys while the children and Gita, now nineteen, played baseball on Adam's Wii and splashed around in the pool. I thought of that sunny Sunday in February when we'd last come here together, about the many unknowns I had yet to face. I thought of our family photo on the boardwalk bench. It felt good to be looking at that day and all of my subsequent suffering through a rearview mirror.

The mood was bittersweet. Everyone wished us well on our impending London adventure, but no one wanted us to go, and they said as much.

"This sucks," Rivky said when we were alone on the balcony.

"I know." I sighed and hugged her tight. "But think of it this way: Had we not decided to go, I would have waited much longer to have my mastectomy and that would have been a disaster." I stopped short of saying that I might be dead by now. It was harsh but true. My cancer had been aggressive and fast-moving. The way I saw it, London saved my life. Sooner or later, I'd have some version of this conversation with anyone who was sad about our departure. My go-to line was, "Alive in London or dead in New Jersey. Which would you prefer?"

For Miryam and Rivky in particular, our move felt like an abandonment. I wished there was a way to reconcile what was best *for* me with what my sisters needed *from* me, but there wasn't. I was the same person who, at twenty, rejected suggestions that I drop out of college to run the household after my mom died. I had a husband and kids of my own to consider and had to do what was best for them. I'd have to find new ways to show up for my sisters from far away.

Gita had finished her gap year and decided to study science at a university in Tel Aviv. She was moving to Israel, essentially, so if anything, our move to London was a plus for her. We'd be a quick four-hour plane ride away.

The past ten months had been emotionally draining on everyone we loved and leaving so soon after felt abrupt. I would have loved to stay another six to twelve months post-treatment so friends and family could see me back on my feet and out of crisis mode. But I was also ready to start afresh someplace where I could talk as much or as little as I chose about what I'd been through; where "cancer" wouldn't be the first thing people thought of when they saw me.

My daily (hourly) inspections of my scalp revealed disappointingly slow progress. Three months post-chemo, I could see the earliest hint of fine, black fuzz starting to peek tentatively out of my hair follicles. This was hardly what I'd pictured when one of my doctors had said "By summer, you'll have hair!"

I arrived at the goodbye party wearing my wig anchored to my head with a Burberry scarf Phil bought me for Mother's Day, but an hour in, I had such an intense hot flash, it felt like Satan himself was grilling burgers on a barbecue made of my internal organs. I slipped into the bathroom, ripped everything off my head, and ran my fuzzy scalp under a cool stream from the faucet. My body temperature regulated and my "hair" now dry, I reached for my wig and after a moment's pause, shoved it in my skirt pocket. I tied the scarf around my bare head. *Screw it*, I thought. My comfort finally won over my vanity and by then, my kids had proven they were oblivious to my quirky hairstyles and accessories. I like to think this was the result of my diligence in keeping them from seeing the scary stuff. I could see a day, way down the road, when I'd tell them everything. I would tell them what an important role they played in saving my life. For now, though, it was a relief to be able to delay that conversation for as long as I needed, until they were older, and when the trauma was far behind me.

The only photo of me wearing a scarf on my bald head and looking like a stereotypical chemo patient was taken when I was no longer a chemo patient. I'm standing next to Phil at the party, leaning into him with my hand on his chest. My smile is the kind that can come only from the relief of a thirty-degree drop in body temperature and from being surrounded by everyone you love in the world: everyone who loves you.

On moving day, Tamar and her kids were the first to arrive and the last to leave. Like me, Tamar has never been quick to cry. We both took pride in our pragmatic approach to life and our stellar coping skills. We saved our tears for when they really mattered, or for when the emotion was so great, even we couldn't hold them back. And now, in my upstairs bathroom, which by the next day would belong to another family—renters who'd signed a two-year lease—I was peeling back the front of my paisley bandana and showing her my downy skull fuzz and she was crying and I was crying.

"It looks cool, Gi, very punk," she said, blowing her nose.

"If it's so cool then *you* do it," I blubbered back, and we laughed despite ourselves.

"I've always wanted to," she said, and the floodgates opened. We both knew we weren't crying about buzzcuts.

We eventually joined what felt like the rest of the neighborhood downstairs. All day long, friends, classmates, and teachers came to say goodbye. My brother brought his kids over and the cousins sat on the floor eating ices and trading Pokémon cards. Hayley caught some of the action on Polaroid and left me with the photos before giving me a hug and a promise to visit soon, even though she'd left the same London neighborhood we were moving to a good many years before. Effy, wanting to beat the crowds and have a private audience with me and Phil, had stopped by the evening before. He and Phil hugged and slapped each other loudly on the back the way men inexplicably do. Then he turned to me.

"Still not too late to change your mind, you know. England sucks." For whatever reason, he'd always hated England and now hated it even more.

"And pass up the chance to force you to visit me there? Never."

"I hope it rains the whole time you're there," he said, only half-jokingly.

I rolled my eyes. "On a serious note, though," I said, "I know I've thanked you for everything, but I'm saying it again. It couldn't have been easy to see me that way and you really stepped up to the plate. You were perfect for the job."

"It was worth it just to see you cry for once," he said, tearing up.

"Well, it looks like we're even now," I said, and we hugged goodbye.

Hayley, Tamar, and a few of their kids stayed until the bitter end, helping us load our suitcases into the van waiting to take us to Newark airport. We hugged again and again as if trying to stock up for scarce times ahead. Ezra, Lea, and Tani said goodbye to their bedrooms, goodbye to the playroom now empty of toys, goodbye to the backyard where they'd skidded down a Slip 'N Slide only the day before. Back outside, Phil was chasing Kivi up and down the driveway. I handed the kids each a piece of jumbo chalk from a bucket on our front porch and told them, "There's a new family coming to stay in our house while we're gone. Let's make them feel welcome!" and in huge blue letters, I wrote "Welcome Home" on the asphalt driveway. Ezra added a yellow turtle. Lea, a pink heart. Tani drew something green and Kivi poked the driveway with his orange chalk, leaving a spray of dots.

We pulled away and I tried to take another series of rapid fire snapshots with my mind, this time of our weeping cherry tree against the backdrop of our wood-shingled house, the basketball hoop, the newly decorated driveway, the wooden front door that I kept varnished to a high shine by adding a coat each year, the cement porch that had held our wooden bench, the one I'd sat on as a bride at our wedding that was repurposed as a delivery and pickup hub for food/books/household supplies and kids' coats left in each other's cars—the bench that was now in a shipping container on its way, as were we, to our new life in London.

12

the mom who knew too much

There was a time, around six months after our move to London, when I came close to telling my kids that I'd had chemotherapy. We were in Jerusalem for winter break in late December 2009, and by then, my hair was around the same length it was when Raluca had cut it. I was sick of wearing a hat and wig constantly, sick of having to keep up my self-imposed masquerade in front of the kids.

Phil and I left the kids with a babysitter one night and went to dinner. On our way to the restaurant, I removed my cap and peeled off the wig, exposing my head to the cool Jerusalem night air. I stuffed the wig to the bottom of my purse and practiced saying, "I decided to try a short haircut, guys, what do you think?" in an easy, breezy voice. In the morning, I delivered my line as the kids looked at me dubiously.

"Why did you do that, Ma?" asked Lea. It was a fair question from a girl who liked to dress up as a princess. She didn't say I looked bad, only that she couldn't fathom why any woman would cut her hair so short.

"You look like a boy," Ezra observed. He wasn't wrong.

"You look like Magda," said Tani, referring to the cleaning lady who came to our house each week. I couldn't argue with him, either.

"Well, do you guys like it?" I asked, and they answered diplomatically: I looked nice, they agreed, but would I please never cut it that short again.

If the time ever came when they suspected my haircut was anything more, I had my response ready: Mommy had taken some strong medicine to keep her healthy. The medicine worked but it also did something funny to Mommy's hair—it made it short. I've been wearing a wig to look more like me. I'm OK now. I've always been OK.

Nine years later, we were still living in London and my kids were now ten, twelve, fourteen, and sixteen years old. Over the years, I'd explained my family history, BRCA1 status, mastectomy and oophorectomy and why I'd had them, but I never told them about the cancer, how close I'd come to disaster. I never let go of that part of my act and the more time that passed, the harder it was to drop the charade. It felt like I'd been holding my breath for a decade.

One day, I got a phone call from Shera Dubitsky, my good friend and the longtime clinical director of Sharsheret, a national nonprofit that supports young Jewish women facing breast cancer. I turned to them for support during my surgeries and treatment. The core of Sharsheret was their link program, aptly named since sharsheret is Hebrew for "chain." A link was like a cancer buddy with personal experience or knowledge about specific aspects of the disease. Whether someone was a BRCA carrier with a family history seeking prevention options, a woman looking to freeze her eggs before starting chemo, or a mother seeking advice on how to talk to her young children about her advanced cancer, there was always a link who'd at one point been in the same boat and could therefore offer meaningful support. Like me, Shera had lost her mother to breast cancer at a young age. And in 2008, Shera became my link—more like my lifeline—and we'd kept in touch long after my ordeal was behind me.

"Hey, Gila," her warm, baritone voice booming through the phone. "I have something important to ask you and you don't have to answer right away, but promise me you'll think about it."

I promised. I couldn't imagine Shera asking for anything I'd ever say no to.

"OK. Would you consider being the keynote speaker at this year's benefit? Your story is so powerful; sharing it with an audience will get them to ramp up their breast health activity for sure!" Sounding as excited as she always was when it came to prevention, Shera was referring to Sharsheret's annual fund-raising brunch, which had been held in a New Jersey hotel every May since its inception.

Before moving to London, I'd never missed a benefit. What started out as an event for around a hundred women quickly grew into one that packed a hotel ballroom with more than six hundred guests each year. Part of my contribution was ~~badgering~~ recruiting friends to attend. I was proud to be closely tied to Sharsheret, in no small part because its founder, Rochelle Shoretz, was my old high school classmate.

When Rochelle was twenty-eight and a mother of two young boys, she found a lump in her breast. She was frustrated by the lack of support available to women as young as she was, so she started Sharsheret from her chemo chair. I immediately got involved as a volunteer doing mailings and outreach and was proud to see it grow into a nationally recognized organization. After seven clean years, her cancer returned, this time Stage IV. It had metastasized all over her body. She passed away at age forty-two, the same age my mom had been.

I considered Shera's request about speaking at the brunch. After all she'd done for me, of course I wanted to say yes, but there was one thing holding me back. I'd have to fly to New Jersey for the event and I couldn't just disappear for a few days without my kids wondering where I'd gone and why.

After taking a few days, I called Shera while sitting in my parked car in the driveway just before school pickup.

"I want to say yes," I told her, "but the problem is that I still haven't told my kids about the cancer part. What if I tell them now, so many years later, and it makes them angry, like 'Mom, why would you keep something like that from us?' Was it a mistake to hide it from them all these years?"

"You're in the waiting room," she said. A clean, blunt metaphor. Classic Shera.

"The what?"

"The waiting room," she repeated. "It's the worst because you're hovering between two worlds. You need closure. Remember when you were waiting for results from a pathology report? What was the worst part? The not knowing. You've been in the waiting room with your kids for so long you've gotten comfortable in your discomfort of *not* telling them. Leaving the waiting room is freaking you out. You'll feel so much better once you're out of it. I promise."

She gave me some excellent tips for talking to each of the kids in age-appropriate, individualized ways.

- Tell them separately.

- Let them ask questions, cry, laugh, or not react at all.

- Answer them honestly and clearly, don't overcomplicate things.

- Don't turn it into a lecture about breast cancer; it's not the right time.

- Give them space to process and be prepared for follow-up questions in the coming days, weeks, months, forever. You never know what nugget of information might embed itself into their brains and dislodge years later as a question needing an answer.

- Tell them you're going to speak at an event full of people to share your story in the hope that it spreads the word and encourages people to take care of their health.

- Count yourself lucky that after all these years, your community has respected your wishes in protecting the kids from knowing about your illness and that you get to be the one to choose just the right words to tell them.

"Call me once you've told them. Good luck, you've got this!" she said.

One Sunday afternoon, a few weeks after that fateful phone call, I sat down on my bed with each of my kids, one at a time, and told them the part of my story they didn't know. I told them, in words carefully chosen to suit their individual ages, about what I'd done to make sure I got to keep doing my favorite thing: being their mom.

Ezra (sixteen) cried a little, not sad tears, but the kind that come when you can't quite find the words you want to say. He gave me an uncharacteristically long hug.

Lea (fourteen): "Wow, Mom, you're my hero!" which made *me* cry.

Tani (twelve) was pensive. "Hunh," he started, and then, "Wait, was that a wig under your hat when we were little?" He'd always been a perceptive child; it was a miracle he never made this observation during my treatment. I told him it was and that I still had it if he ever wanted to see it. He declined.

Kivi (ten), too young to remember what I looked like all those years ago, just gave me a hug and told me he was proud of me.

I sat on my bed for a long time after Kivi left, awash in a sea of endorphins and wondering why I'd tortured myself by sitting in the waiting room for so long. The last time I felt such ecstatic relief was when I woke up from an eight-hour surgery and my breasts were gone.

I called Shera the next day.

"I told them. It went great. Your advice was perfect," I said, before adding, "I'll do it. I'll be a Sharsheret honoree this May."

"Wooohooo!" she cheered before making another request. "Your story is super impactful on its own, but as a family, you'll really blow people's minds. Do you think you might convince your sisters to join you?"

When I first told Miryam and Rivky about my decision to undergo a double mastectomy, they were as supportive and encouraging as any big sister could hope for. They were clear, however, that they would not take such drastic measures themselves. That Thanksgiving phone call from my surgeon rocked their worlds as much as it did mine. It plucked breast cancer out of the past and slung it right in front of their faces, daring them to do something about it. Shortly after my diagnosis, Miryam and Rivky went for genetic testing. Both were, unsurprisingly, BRCA positive and both went on to have preventative double mastectomies in their twenties.

Rivky, only twenty-four at the time of my diagnosis, already mother to an adorable little girl and expecting another, waited a few more years and had another baby before opting for the same procedure Miryam had (with implants for reconstruction rather than a TRAM Flap like I'd had) in order to be able to have more kids post-mastectomy.

To say I was proud of them is an understatement. They sensed a clear and present danger and, instead of hiding, took an aggressive stance and got ahead of it, just like I did. I was far from a perfect sister, coming up short in so many ways, especially during the years when I was away at college and working. I tried hard to balance showing up both for them and for myself. Perhaps my diagnosis was the ultimate way of showing up, like throwing myself on a grenade and sparing them from its impact. The vow I'd whispered in my mother's ear when she had minutes left to live had been a hard one to keep: "Don't worry about the kids; I promise I'll look after them." Finally, I felt that I was honoring my words.

Miryam agreed to be my co-honoree at the Sharsheret fundraiser; Rivky, our more private sister, said she'd cheer us on from the sidelines.

The morning of the fundraiser arrived. Miryam and I took our places at the podium on the ballroom stage. Over six hundred people, mainly women in vibrant, floral dresses, sat at round tables that reached from one end of the room to the next, enjoying a brunch of salads, sea bass, and quiches ("mom food," as my kids would call it). Phil's mother, aunt, and Grandma GG sat at a table close to the stage. Rivky and Eli sat with them, too. I only wished Gita could have been there, but Tel Aviv was a twelve-hour flight away. Lots of our friends came to show their support including Stephanie, my original inspiration for my double mastectomy. Tamar, Hayley, and Effy showed me mercy by sitting far enough back that I couldn't see them once the house lights went down. If I made eye contact with any one of them, I doubt I'd have been able to stop my tears.

Phil and I had agreed he'd stay back in London with the kids. Ideally they'd have been in that room with me, but we didn't want to interrupt their school week or deal with the jet lag.

In the run-up to the event, Miryam and I decided against giving two separate speeches. It would be more impactful to speak in tandem, passing the baton back and forth to demonstrate how intertwined our stories of prevention and survival were.

Moments before we began, my friend Adina, for whom I'd served as a Sharsheret link, offered to livestream our speech.

"Is that a thing?" I asked, excited by the prospect of Phil and the kids tuning in live.

"Yeah, Instagram has a 'live' feature now, didn't you know?" I did not. I texted Phil about this development and handed her my phone. She moved to a seat closer to the stage to get a better angle.

At the podium, Miryam and I stood shoulder to shoulder, surreptitiously adjusting our microphones way down to suit our height. My mouth was bone-dry, my heart galloping. Even with my sister next to me, I was nervous and very grateful when the room went dark, and the blinding spotlights obscured the crowd. Miryam, a seasoned public speaker, began and I waited for my cue to jump in. Staring into the void, I directed my words to a remote audience of five. I pictured them watching on Phil's iPhone screen many miles away. I spoke as though I was addressing only them. For all of the times my kids turned a deaf ear to my incessant directives to flush the toilet, pick their socks up off the floor, and soak their dishes after eating mac and cheese, I knew they were listening now.

As we moved through our story of sick parents, loss, and taking control of our health while rebuilding our family from scratch, all we could hear were the soft sighs, the clicking of tongues, and tearful sniffles of a rapt audience. To alleviate the tension, we threw in a few jokes about the advantages of being short (saving money by shopping in the kids' department, for one). The relief was palpable.

We finished to thunderous applause followed by an avalanche of hugs, and when I was finally able to sneak away to a quiet corner outside the ballroom, I called Phil. The kids were all yelling into the phone, "Great job, Ma! You were so good, I'm proud of you!" and "Your makeup looks awesome!" (Lea) and "Do they have cookies with logos printed on them? Bring some of those home, please, Mom" (Tani).

"I love you guys so much," I said, my voice catching.

Twenty-six years had passed since that day at JFK airport when my mother laid her fears at my feet. Whether or not it was fair, I felt back then it was too much to ask me to carry. Her cancer, I believed, could have been avoided or at least survived. Now I stood near a floor-to-ceiling window, gazing out past the full hotel parking lot as I held my phone—my precious children's voices—to my ear. Not only had I survived, but here were my kids celebrating my survival. The difference between their experience and mine was night and day. It was stunning. My mother's legacy to me was a resolve to avoid breast cancer at all costs. In response to how she dealt with her risk and subsequent illness, I developed a fierce commitment to protecting my kids from trauma. I could hold ten times the terror in my heart if it meant leaving them with none.

The first inkling my kids had that their mom ever had cancer came when the threat was way in the past. By the time they learned the truth, I'd undergone the surgeries, had the chemo, and went through menopause. It took more than three years, but my hair finally grew back to its normal length. Every turn, every step on my path to prevention followed my four children who served as my North Star. I did everything to give them what my eighteen-year-old-self needed but was denied. I never knew—never asked—how my grandmother had spoken to my young mother about her own illness and her imminent death. I wonder if they ever spoke about it at all. My instinct to buffer my kids from trauma, comes, of course, from having had no buffer from my own. My hope is to leave them with a better legacy than the one I inherited. If in some parallel universe my mother is reading this, I want her to know that I'm sorry she didn't have any buffers, either. I think that maybe she did the best she could with what little resources she had. I want her to know that even though it came at a very high price, she instilled me with life-saving lessons, which I'll pass down to my own kids. And for that, I am so thankful.

CUSTOMER SATISFACTION SURVEY

We know that when it comes to universes, you've got lots of options (particularly since the introduction of the Multiverse!), so we appreciate you choosing us, This Universe™! Our aim at This Universe™ is to ensure the growth, progress, comfort, and joy (tempered with adversity) of our clientele. Our customer care team has taken notice of your freakish ability to sidestep some of the challenges we send your way, a clear indication that you're not entirely satisfied with what we have in store for you. Your feedback is important to us. We ask that you take a few moments to complete this survey so that we can tailor our offers accordingly.

Being from Staten Island: 3/5 stars

Until recently, I'd have given it one star (or zero, if that was an option) but time, distance, and Pete Davidson have softened my perspective. I now look back fondly on the warm, sheltered (and stinky) years spent cut off from pretty much the rest of the world in my early childhood. An added bonus: It gives me street cred at dinner parties.

Growing up without cable TV: 0/5 stars

Were you waiting for me to say that I'm a more wholesome, enriched individual having gone through my adolescence without MTV or HBO? Well, I'm not. My pop education is stunted and I still, as a woman nearing the age of fifty, have to play catch up. I would have liked to have gone to school knowing all the dance moves to Janet

Jackson's *Rhythm Nation* like my friends did. It was the equivalent of a kid today growing up without the internet. Pass.

Standing at my parents' bedsides as they took their last breaths: 5/5 stars

The five-star rating may come as a surprise, but hear me out. It was an honor and a privilege to be present as each of my parents left this world. Not everyone has that opportunity.

It was a final chance to uphold the most important commandment—to honor your father and mother—while they were still alive.

Menopause at thirty-five: 2/5 stars

This experience can vary greatly from person to person so if you've had early menopause, I'd love to hear how it went for you! It was difficult to tell whether my hot flashes, mood swings, and poor sleep were related to the abrupt ending of my period or the stress of moving to another country with four little kids, but I counted myself lucky to be so distracted that I couldn't wallow in the symptoms. The dip in estrogen also impacted my bone density, so I have to stave off osteoporosis with medication. As for my period stopping, that's been pretty great, if I'm being honest.

One whole star comes from my vantage point as a middle-aged woman now watching my friends in the throes of their own extreme hormonal fluctuations and nodding my head sympathetically while high-fiving myself for having gotten all that out of the way years before.

Having a double mastectomy five years before Angelina Jolie made it popular: 5/5 stars

Look, it's never fun when a celebrity copies you and takes credit for your idea, but Angelina made it much easier for me to get the word out about prevention. She saves me a lot of time having to explain what kind of surgery I had; all I have to say is "You know the one Angelina Jolie had? That's what I did. But I did it *first.*"

Being a mom: 5/5 stars (my kids might be reading this)

Being a mother is a deeply profound experience full of surprises. Kids are born with inherent personalities and they're you but also not you and it's humbling and frustrating and definitely not for everyone, but it is very much for me. Of all the job titles I've held in the past, and whatever I go on to accomplish in the future, the role I identify with the most is "Mom." The parameters of my job constantly shift but the title remains constant. And if you're my kid and reading this—wow, you made it all the way to the end of my book!

Having it all: N/A

I can't rate something that never existed in the first place. That phrase should be outlawed.

Starting your day with gratitude: 5/5 stars

Stop rolling your eyes and just try it, OK?

Being an oldest sibling: 4.5/5 stars

Awesome, highly recommend. Loses half a star because of that time one of my sisters said, "I feel bad for you. You don't have you for a big sister." Before then I'd never thought how great it would have been to have someone pave the way for me, someone to look up to. I get sad about it once in a blue moon. But mostly, being the oldest rocks.

Having an overactive imagination: 4/5 stars

I am never ever bored. My mind churns out scenarios, exaggerates reality, plays a 24-7 game of "what-if" on a constant loop. As a result, I can be very entertaining not only to others but to myself, too. My overactive imagination loses a star for the exhaustion it causes me and the inability to control myself from conjuring outlandish worst-case scenarios. I've also heard this referred to as "anxiety." I'm looking into it.

General anesthesia: 5/5 stars

Utterly delightful. Worth the few days of brain fog, sore throat, and excessive gas.

Marrying a guy because he shares a birthday with your dead mother: 5/5 stars

Disclaimer: I am by no means endorsing this practice, I'm just saying it really worked out for me.

Aging: 5/5 stars

I don't care how saggy, dumpy, wrinkly, gray, thick-waisted, brittle-boned, sleep deprived, vison impaired, hard of hearing, constipated, nose hair-sprouting, creaky-jointed, dentally challenged, arthritis riddled you get. Aging beats the alternative, end of story.

Cemeteries: 3/5 stars

Very grounding (see what I did there?). Peaceful. Acceptable to shun small talk no matter how many people you run into there, although the number of people you run into are minimal, which definitely earns cemeteries a star. I didn't give them five stars because there's too much pressure to feel something, to connect with your dearly departed in a specific place. My mother is in the scent of brisket filling my kitchen each Friday when I cook for Shabbat. She's in the centerpieces I handmade for my kids' bar and bat mitzvahs because why pay for something you can make yourself? The sound of a spoon tinkling against a coffee mug conjure memories of my father, and I see his face when my boys wrap their arms in the leather straps of tefillin before praying, just like he did.

Sarcasm: 8/5 stars
Sometimes even my closest friends aren't sure if I'm being earnest or sarcastic and that is my superpower.

Wigs: 5/5 stars
Religious implications aside, wigs provide dignity and confidence to women, children, and men alike who experience hair loss for whatever reason. I applaud and am very much in awe of people who choose to put their baldness on public display, but for me, cranial prostheses were integral to my survival.

Writing a memoir: 0/5 stars
Draining. Gut wrenching. Self-doubt sowing. Insanity inducing. Time sucking. Eyeball burning. Wrist destroying. Also back, neck, shoulders, and ass destroying. All consuming. The worst. Whose stupid idea was this anyway? Do not do this. Avoid at all costs.

Publishing a memoir: 5/5 stars
I'm still not advising that you do this, but man it feels good to hold your book in your hands and see the story that, for years, has been screeching around inside you like a banshee finally expunged, out in the world, no longer buzzing nonstop in your ear to tell it tell it *tell it*. Just tell your story already, dammit.

acknowledgments

Whenever I pick up a book, the first thing I read is the Acknowledgements. It's a peek into the author's inner world and a reminder of just how many people it took to bring their book into existence. As a debut author who's been saying "I'm going to write a memoir!" for more than a decade, I'm so lucky to have a long list of people to thank for getting *Nearly Departed* out into the world. Less lucky for you if you don't enjoy reading long lists.

Myrsini Stephanides: You had me at "wickedly funny." Thank you for understanding exactly what I'm trying to say even when I do not. Batya Rosenblum: You found the arc in my narrative and brought this story in for a landing. I couldn't ask for a more bashert editor. Thanks to Beth Bugler for designing the cover of my dreams, Matthew Lore for taking a chance on this newbie author, Besse Lynch for publicity, Zach Pace, Ally Mitchell, and Juliann Barbato.

Leigh Stein: You laid your hands over mine and helped me shape this story into something real, like the pottery scene in *Ghost* but with a book. Erin Niumata: Thank you for your friendship, years of guidance, and believing in me from the start.

I'm so lucky to be part of a community of writers who are also my friends. Whether you were an early reader, my teacher, cheerleader, or ass kicker, your contributions were essential and have made all the difference. Wendi Aarons, Caitlin Kunkel, Dana Jeri Maier, Lea Goldman (the original Shabbos Queen), Dina Gachman, Kate Rosow Chrisman (who cared about my book as if it was her own), Sarah Cottrell, Rebecca Morrison, Lyndsay Rush (aka Mary Oliver's Drunk Cousin), Jen Mann, Emi Nietfeld, Rax King, Amy Shearn, Ely Kreimendahl, Andrea Guevara, Rachel Sobel. I hope I get the chance to reciprocate some day!

Abby Alten Schwartz, Nikki Campo, Amy Paturel, LaVonne Roberts and Helen Wolkowicz: Your love and support are palpable from many time zones away.

Thanks to my creative friends Rachael Kay Albers, Tara Clark, Terri Fry, Priscilla Kavanaugh, and Aliette Silva for letting me vent weekly. Special thanks to Priscilla for feedback on my manuscript.

Lucy Huber and Christopher Monks: Thank you for publishing the piece I'm most proud of writing in McSweeney's, "An Open Letter to Tiffany & Co. About Their Advertising Campaign for the Ring that Helps Women Remember They Survived Cancer."

Thanks to my London friends for your input and for getting me out of my own way: Katherine Buckle Humphries, my elegant voice of reason, Athena Giannaros, my Greek goddess with a Jewish heart, Kerry Rosenfeld, my dark-humored partner in crime, Chagit Blass, my Jewish Wikipedia. Thanks to Ayelet Garson for waving your magic wand over my face and hair for my photo shoots.

And my friends who go back further: Tamar Loheit, Hayley Faber, Chani Roth, Effy Zinkin for letting me dig into your brains and scoop out memories with melon ballers; they added depth and clarity to my storytelling. Stephanie Bulgar-Brooks, my fellow Capricorn, Cindy Henzel for reading speedily and with an open heart, Shari Teigman as well as George and Miriam Teigman z"l: you know why. Shera Dubitsky and everyone at Sharsheret for having all the time in the world for me. Ingrid Davies: thanks for brushing the dust off of old memories. I'm happy this book brought you back into my life.

Shital Patel for fixing my wrecked back every other week only for me to wreck it again by hunching over a keyboard for hours at a time.

To any friends who made the grave mistake of asking me how my book was coming along, only to find yourselves trapped in a twenty-minute rant about edits, deadlines, manuscripts, word count, and my chronic back pain: Thank you for listening; it lightened my burden.

Miryam, Rivky, and Gita: Sisters by birth, but friends by ch– no, I can't, it's too cheesy. Thank you for helping me remember and for reading excerpts and chapters over and over. I love you, mine *shvesters*.

To my wonderful children, whose culinary skills improved dramatically when I stopped cooking dinner for a year:

Ezra for incorporating the phrase "The Mom Who Knew Too Much" into every conversation.

Lea for being my very own, real-life cheerleader (complete with uniform) and early reader.

Tani for breaking up long nights at my desk with *Family Guy* clips to make me laugh.

Kivi for peeking into my office each night before you went to bed and asking how the writing was going, then giving me a thumbs-up. Those thumbs-ups sustained me. I love you guys so much.

Phil: Thank you for your unwavering love and support and for reminding me to guardrail my time in order to write this book, even when that meant a sharp decline in my attention to household responsibilities. To paraphrase George McFly in *Back to the Future*: You are my density.

about the author

GILA PFEFFER is a Jewish American humor writer and personal essayist whose work has appeared in McSweeney's, *The New York Times*, *The New Yorker*, Today.com, and elsewhere. Gila's "Feel It on the First" campaign uses tongue-in-cheek photo and video reminders to prioritize breast health, which have directly led to earlier diagnoses and treatment for some very grateful women. She splits her time between New York City and London. *Nearly Departed* is her first book.

gilapfeffer.com | ⓞ gilapfeffer